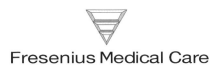

Good Nephrological Practice

Management of the Renal Patient: Clinical Algorithms on Vascular Access for Haemodialysis

Editors

Ali Bakran

Volker Mickley

Jutta Passlick-Deetjen

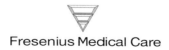

Fresenius Medical Care

Library of Congress Cataloging-in-Publication Data

Bakran, Ali / Mickley, Volker / Passlick-Deetjen, Jutta:
Management of the Renal Patient: Clinical Algorithms on Vascular Access for Haemodialysis. – Lengerich; Berlin; Bremen; Miami; Riga; Viernheim; Wien; Zagreb: Pabst Science Publishers, 2003

2nd Edition
ISBN 3-936142-86-6

This work is subject to copyright. All rights are reserved, whether the whole or part of the material is concerned, specifically the rights of translation, reprinting, reuse of illustrations, recitation, broadcasting, reproduction on microfilms or in other ways, and storage in data banks. The use of registered names, trademarks, etc. in this publication does not imply, even in the absence of a specific statement, that such names are exempt from the relevant protective laws and regulations and therefore free for general use.

Medicine is an ever-changing science. As new research and clinical experience broaden our knowledge, changes in treatment and drug therapy are required. The editors and members of the Medical Expert Group have checked with sources believed to be reliable in their efforts to provide information and have created algorithms that are generally in accord with the standards accepted at the time of publication. In view of the possibility of human error or changes in medical knowledge, neither the editors nor the publisher or any other party who has been involved in the preparation or publication of this work warrants that the information contained herein is in every respect accurate or complete, and they are not responsible for any errors or omissions or the results obtained from the use of such information. Readers are encouraged to confirm the information contained herein with other sources.

Printed and bound by:
mt druck Walter Thiele GmbH & Co., D-63263 Neu-Isenburg
www.mt-druck.de

Published by:
Pabst Science Publishers, D-49525 Lengerich
www.pabst-publishers.com

ISBN 3-936142-86-6

Clinical Algorithms on Vascular Access for Haemodialysis

Editors:
Ali Bakran, FRCS (The Royal Liverpool University Hospital, United Kingdom)
Volker Mickley, M.D. (Stadtklinik Baden-Baden, Germany)
Prof. Jutta Passlick-Deetjen, M.D. (Fresenius Medical Care Deutschland GmbH, Germany)

Medical Expert Group:
Prof. Bernard Canaud, M.D. (Hôpital Lapeyronie, Montpellier, France)
Patrick Haage, M.D. (University of Technology, Aachen, Germany)
Joerg Hoffmann, M.D. (Fresenius Medical Care Deutschland GmbH, Germany)
Klaus Konner, M.D. (Merheim Hospital, University of Cologne, Germany)
Pedro Ponce, M.D. (Hospital Garcia d' Orta, Pragal, Portugal)
Jeffrey J. Sands, M.D. (Fresenius Medical Care North America, USA)
Jan H. M. Tordoir, M.D. (University Hospital, Maastricht, The Netherlands)

Revised and Endorsed by the Council of the Vascular Access Society

President:
Ali Bakran (The Royal Liverpool University Hospital, Liverpool, UK)

Council Members:
Joaquim Barbosa (Hospital Particular de Lisboa, Lisbon, Portugal)
Pierre Bourquelot (Clinique Jouvenet, Paris, France)
Salvatore Di Giulio (Hospital San Camillo Forlanini, Rome, Italy)
Miltos K. Lazarides (Demokritos University of Thrace, Alexandroupolis, Greece)
Marko Malovrh (University Medical Centre, Ljubljana, Slovenia)
Volker Mickley (Stadtklinik Baden-Baden, Germany)
Josette Pengloan (Centre Hospitalier Universitaire, Tours, France)
Jose R. Polo (Hospital Universitario Gregorio Maranon, Madrid, Spain)
Jan H. M. Tordoir (University Hospital, Maastricht, The Netherlands)
Luc Turmel-Rodrigues (Clinique St-Gatien, Tours, France)
Dierk Vorwerk (Klinikum Ingolstadt, Germany)

Scientific Secretary:
Alexandra Reber (Fresenius Medical Care Deutschland GmbH, Germany)

CONTENTS

Foreword 9
Introduction 11
Symbols and abbreviations 12
Glossary 13

1. Starting Management of Vascular Access 15
2. Patient with Acute Need for Dialysis Access 18
3. Clinical Evaluation of Access Site 21
4. Placement of Forearm A/V Fistula 26
5. Placement of Elbow or Upper Arm A/V Fistula 32
6. Placement of Graft 36
7. Placement and Routine Management of Tunneled Catheter .. 41
8. Postoperative Control of A/V Fistula and Graft Function (1) .. 46
9. Postoperative Control of A/V Fistula and Graft Function (2) .. 49
10. Routine Management of A/V Fistula and Graft 52
11. Identification of A/V Fistula and Graft Problems 58
12. Management of A/V Fistula Stenosis 64
13. Management of A/V Fistula Thrombosis 67
14. Management of Autogenous A/V Fistula Infection
    after 1st Month of Placement 70
15. Management of Graft Stenosis 73
16. Management of Graft Thrombosis 76
17. Management of Graft Infection After 1st Month of Placement (1) .. 80
18. Management of Graft Infection After 1st Month of Placement (2) .. 83
19. Management of Aneurysms 85
20. Management of High Flow in A/V Fistula and Graft 87
21. Management of Ischaemia (1) 89
22. Management of Ischaemia (2) 92
23. Management of Central Venous Obstruction (1) 95
24. Management of Central Venous Obstruction (2) 98
25. Identification and Management of Tunneled Catheter
    Complications 101
26. Management of Tunneled Catheter Infection 105

Appendix I: Diagnostics 109
Appendix II: Vascular Access Creation 113
Appendix III: Monitoring 117
Appendix IV: Treatment of Stenosis and Thrombosis 120
Appendix V: Vascular Access Infections in Dialysis Patients .. 125

References 128

Foreword by the President of the Vascular Access Society

Vascular access is absolutely critical to the well being and survival of the patient requiring haemodialysis and yet is often badly supported. The Vascular Access Society was established to improve the status and quality of vascular access performance by encouraging good practice. It was felt that there was insufficient provision both nationally and internationally for this very important aspect of patient care and need. Our young Society has already made a significant contribution to improving knowledge amongst surgeons, nephrologists, radiologists, dialysis nurses and other healthcare workers about vascular access by organising courses and congresses. The Society considers this extension into the development of guidelines in vascular access management and care, as a natural step forward. The guidelines take a problem-based approach and are meant to help the healthcare professional in a comprehensive and schematic manner in every day practice. It is not a book to read but, rather, a reference for those facing practical problems, to delve into and seek guidance. Common problems are covered by logical, step by step algorithms and the investigations and management recommended on the basis of best evidence. Unfortunately, the evidence-base of vascular access is often sparse since there are too few randomised controlled trials. Nevertheless, recommendations have been made from the wealth of collective experience of the nephrologists, radiologists and surgeons who have together helped to draw up the algorithms.

Needless to say any advice given must be interpreted in the local clinical context. The vascular access needs of individual patients requires flexibility and adjustment to local circumstances. Clinical practice is always a compromise between what is ideal and what local conditions will allow. In principle, however, we feel that the guidelines offer current best practice. The emphasis remains on the benefits of autogenous A/V fistula over grafts, the creation of fistulas during the pre-dialysis period to avoid use of dialysis catheters, and, particularly, the importance of a multidisciplinary approach to problem management.

Ali Bakran
President of the Vascular Access Society
Consultant Transplant and Vascular Surgeon
The Royal Liverpool University Hospital

Introduction

Vascular access management is central to maintain patients' health and quality to life. For this reason we feel that it is important to provide an easily used reference including sections on vascular access planning, placement, and treatment of access complications. Although these subjects have been covered in the DOQI[1] and K/DOQI[2] it is important to have an European document, which reflects European practices and experience. These are very different from the United States perspective with their heavy reliance on grafts and catheters. We also wish to make this a living document that is practical both for reference and for use in the day to day management of patients. It is broken down into a sequence of algorithms, which link together in succeeding sections. Each algorithm has numerical links to the text, which explain and provide data, evidence and references to support each branch of the decision tree. It is our hope that his can serve as resource for caregivers and patients at all levels of expertise. With this in mind, we will begin an integrated approach to access management starting with the conservative treatment of chronic renal insufficiency, gradually progressing to the need for haemodialysis, either directly or via PD or transplantation. Underlining this document is the philosophy of preventing complications by maximizing use of A/V fistulas and by having fistulas available, commencing with the very first dialysis. This avoidance of catheters and reliance on A/V fistulas ensures the best clinical outcomes with the fewest complications.

Jeffrey Sands

References:
1. Schwab SJ, Besarab, et al. 1997 525 /id
2. III. NKF-K/DOQI Clinical Practice Guidelines for Vascular Access: update 2000–2001 14/id

Vascular Access for Haemodialysis Patients
Symbols used for the Clinical Algorithms

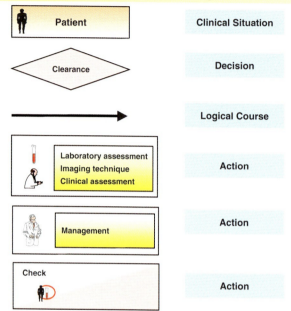

Abbreviations

AAI	Arm – arm index	h	Hour(s)
AB	Antibiotics	HD	Haemodialysis
ASA	American Society of Anesthesiologists	IU	International units
A/V	Arterio-venous	i.v.	Intravenous
BP	Blood pressure	MAP	Mean arterial pressure
BMI	Body mass index	max.	Maximum
CABG	Coronary artery bypass graft	min.	Minimum
CCr	Creatinine clearance	mon	Month(s)
CFU	Colony forming units	MRA	Magnetic resonance angiography
CHF	Chronic heart failure	MRSA	Methicillin resistant staphylococcus aureus
cm	Centimetre	PAOD	Peripheral arterial occlusive disease
CRI	Chronic renal insufficiency	PD	Peritoneal dialysis
CRP	C-reactive protein	PTA	Percutaneous transluminal angioplasty
CRF	Chronic renal failure	PTFE	Polytetrafluoroethylene
d	Day(s)	Q_a	Vascular access blood flow
dBP	Diastolic blood pressure	Q_b	Extracorporeal blood flow
DOQI	Dialysis Outcomes Quality Initiative	RC	Radio-cephalic
DRIL	Distal revascularization, interval ligation	S. aureus	Staphylococcus aureus
DSA	Digital subtraction angiography	sBP	Systolic blood pressure
DVP	Dynamic venous pressure	SPR	Static venous pressure ratio
ePTFE	expanded Polytetrafluoroethylene	SVP	Static venous pressure
EBPG	European Best Practice Guidelines	tPA	Tissue plasminogen activator
ESRD	End stage renal disease	WBC	White blood cell count
GFR	Glomerular filtration rate	wk	Week(s)
		y	Year(s)

Glossary

A/V fistula	= Autologous arteriovenous access: Haemodialysis access created by direct artery-to-vein anastomosis. Arterial inflow site is reported first, before the venous outflow site (e.g. brachio-cephalic = brachial artery to cephalic vein).
Graft	= Nonautologous arteriovenous access Haemodialysis access created by artery-to-vein interposition of prosthetic conduit (e.g. PTFE or Dacron) or biograft (e.g. bovine heterograft).
Transposition	Peripheral portion of the vein is moved from its original position and connected to the artery, the more central portion of the vein remains intact in its native location.
Translocation	A vein is removed from its origin and is placed in a new place, thus requiring anastomoses to both the arterial and venous segment of the access.
Tunneled	Catheters placed through a subcutaneous tunnel. In general intended for long-term use.
Non-Tunneled	Catheters without a tunnel. In general placed for short term use.
(Non-)Cuffed	Catheters with (without) a subcutaneous cuff.
Patency rate	Percentage of vascular accesses, that remain patent. However, most studies do not use the same definitions and criteria for calculating the patency rate at a given time point, which makes comparison very difficult or even impossible.

Primary patency: Interval between access placement and first intervention or access failure.

Assisted primary patency: Interval between access and first thrombosis. To ensure patency in a still functioning access interventions may be performed during this time interval.

Secondary patency: Total interval from access placement until definite access failure. Interventions for access thrombosis or other complications may be performed during this time interval.

Functional patency: Percentage of vascular accesses, that can be used for haemodialysis and deliver sufficient blood flows.

(For further explanation see publication by Sidawy et al.*)

---

* Sidawy A. N., Gray R., Recommended standards for reports dealing with arteriovenous haemodialysis accesses. J Vasc Surg 2002: 603-610.

Overview of Algorithm Sequence

Placement and Routine Management of Vascular Access:

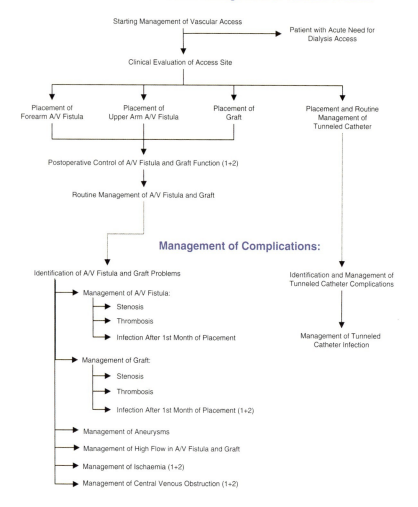

Management of Complications:

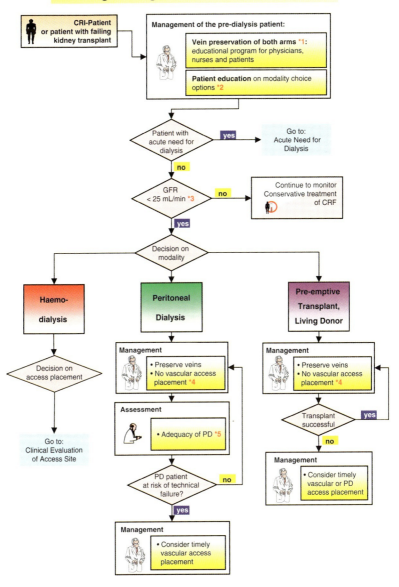

Starting Management of Vascular Access

*1 **Vein preservation of both arms:**
- Veins must be preserved in all patients with declining renal function[1, 2] and those undergoing renal replacement therapy with haemodialysis, peritoneal dialysis and renal transplantation:
  - Avoid i.v. infusion or venipuncture in forearm and upper arm veins of both arms whenever possible.
  - Whenever a central venous catheter is needed, the placement of a subclavian vein catheter must be avoided, as it is usually complicated by subclavian vein stenosis, which has serious implications for future vascular access of HD patients[3]. Catheterisation of the internal jugular or femoral vein is always preferred, although any dialysis catheter can cause central vein stenosis and should be avoided if possible.
  - The patient's vessels should be examined early in the course of chronic renal failure and the best vein for an A/V fistula indicated to the patient so that he/she can prevent use of that vein by healthcare professionals.
  - If the patient is hospitalised: Place sign "no venipuncture" over his or her bed.
  - Consider handing out a "Medic Alert bracelet or card" to the patient.
- Preferred site for venipuncture are the dorsal veins of both hands.
- Educational programmes alerting physicians, nurses and patients of the importance of vein preservation and training in patients with chronic renal failure should be implemented. The programmes should be primarily focused on the patients themselves, who they can contact in the renal outpatient clinic and through their patients' associations. However, these programmes should also address renal physicians and nurses, and staff in the emergency and intensive care units.
- Some believe in vein training although there is no evidence that it is of benefit. For those who do believe in it, vein training can be included into this educational programme. A blood pressure cuff or tourniquet is inflated around the upper arm proximally to the prospective access site, and venous congestion maintained for two or three minutes. This exercise should be repeated several times within a 15 minute period, and the exercise performed three or four times a day. There is no data in the literature on the effect of vein training on vessel diameters and immediate patency rates of newly constructed fistulae. Vein training, however, is believed to further alert the patient on the importance of vein preservation and hence some renal healthcare professionals recommend it.

*2 **Patient education on modality choice options**
- Haemodialysis (HD), peritoneal dialysis (PD) and kidney transplantation all have their place in renal replacement therapy as an integrated therapy approach for ESRD patients. Early patient education should cover all these treatment modalities. There is increasing evidence that early transplantation prolongs life of patients in renal failure and pre-emptive live donor transplantation should be encouraged.
- Early referral to nephrologists may help in decreasing the rate of progression of renal insufficiency and also offers the possibility of timely A/V fistula placement, when needed.
- Educational programmes should involve the entire nephrological team including physicians, surgeons, transplant co-ordinators, nurses, dieticians and social

- workers, and be supported by educational materials such as booklets, flip charts and videos.
- Talking with other patients or visiting haemodialysis or peritoneal dialysis units can help patients prepare and choose the most appropriate modality of treatment.
- In patients who are able and motivated to perform PD, this modality may be the first-line therapy of an integrated therapy approach. In one publication, patients who initially started on PD and were later transferred to HD showed a better survival compared to those started directly on HD[4]. In addition, vascular access sites can be preserved for a later stage in the life of the patient.
- Jungers et al. reported that patients who obtained education over six months prior to initiating dialysis had a significantly shorter length of hospital stay (4.8 + 3.3 days versus 29.7 + 15.8 days), lower three month mortality (1.6% versus 7.1%) and a higher prevalence of home or self care dialysis (40.8% versus 20.1%) than patients referred less than 15 days prior to initiation of dialysis therapy[5].

*3 **GFR < 25 to 20 mL/min**
- When GFR has fallen to below 25 to 20 ml/min the patient, supported by the nephrological team, should decide about the best modality. Irrespectively of the choice of dialysis modality, the forearm and upper arm veins should be preserved for future vascular access surgery. Patients with a GFR < 25–20 ml/min and who have chosen haemodialysis as renal replacement therapy should be seen by a surgeon well-trained in vascular access surgery, within 6 to 12 months of anticipated need for dialysis. Timely consultation with such a vascular access surgeon may markedly reduce the placement of acute catheters for the start of dialysis in favour of fistulas and grafts[1, 6].

*4 **No vascular access placement in PD and kidney transplanted patients**
- Pre-emptive vascular access placement for patients in peritoneal dialysis or renal transplantation is not indicated as the vascular access may never be needed (in more than 90% of cases) and will destroy veins. Moreover, the back-up vascular access often occludes before HD becomes necessary[7].

*5 **Adequacy of PD**
- In PD patients dialysis dose (weekly Kt/V and creatinine clearance) and fluid management should be regularly monitored and adjusted, if necessary, according to the current recommendations of dose, of hydration and cardiovascular status of the patient, respectively[8]. If dialysis dose or ultrafiltration adjustments impose problems a timely planned transfer to HD is recommended. This integrated approach has been shown to improve the patient's survival[4].

References see p. 128

Patient with Acute Need for Dialysis Access

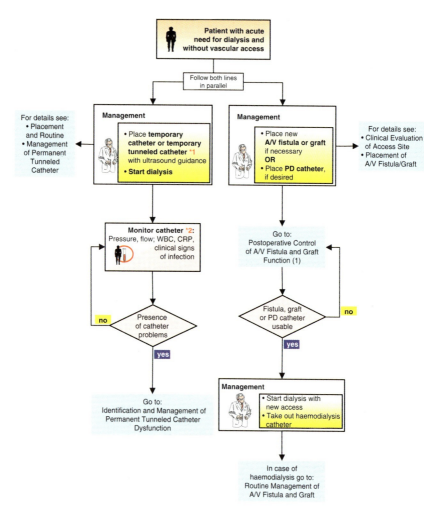

Patient with Acute Need for Dialysis Access

*1 **Place temporary catheter**
- Haemodialysis vascular access catheters are at high risk of infection, thrombosis and other complications[1]. However in emergency cases, they are essential to enable dialysis. Depending on the predicted duration that the catheter is needed, two different kinds of catheters can be used:

a) Catheter placement for up to 2 weeks

Temporary or acute catheters are used in three settings: in patients with acute renal failure, for "in and out" use in patients with temporary loss of permanent access and in critically ill, bed-bound patients[2]. Blood flow ranges from 200–250 ml/min[1] to almost 350 ml/min[2]. For temporary use, soft catheters should be preferred because they are believed to be less traumatic to the vessel wall. The choice between silicone and one of the new polyurethanes is still unresolved.

The femoral route should be the preferred site in an emergency in order to preserve the thoracic venous system. Femoral catheters can be left in place for at least one week. Reported success rates for femoral vein catheterisation are in the range of 95-100 % in patients with palpable femoral arterial pulses[3]. In prospective studies the mean duration of placement was 1 week for temporary polyurethane catheters[3, 4] if ambulation was allowed[4]. The incidence of bacteraemia was 5.4 % after 3 weeks of placement in the internal jugular vein and 10.7 % after one week in the femoral vein[5]. The risk of iliofemoral vein thrombosis may be high: tube-shaped thrombi were detected with colour-coded duplex-ultrasound in 95.7 % cases in a study with a mean catheter dwell time of 17.9 +/-11.2 days[6]. There are no data reported for temporary soft silicone catheters.

b) Catheter placement for more than 2 weeks

Tunneled cuffed catheters should be inserted in situations when the catheter access is required for more than 2 weeks. Thus they may be preferred to bridge the period until an A/V fistula has matured, until a PD catheter can be used or until an anticipated living-related donor transplantation is performed. Finally, they are used as a last resort in patients with no possibility of other dialysis access.

- The right internal jugular vein should be preferred to the left internal jugular vein and to the subclavian veins (see Algorithm: Placement and Routine Management of Tunneled Catheter, *4). It is also possible to use the femoral vein for tunneled cuffed catheters, in order to preserve the central venous system.
- In the case of unexpected long access maturation time, due to borderline quality of the vessels, a decision has to be taken on an individual basis, as to whether the catheter should be used for several weeks or even months, whether the patients should be treated by CAPD during maturation, or whether an AV graft fistula is the better alternative.

*2 **Monitor catheter**
- Temporary and Tunneled cuffed catheters should be monitored clinically for adequate blood-flow delivery, occlusion and potential infection at each treatment. Pre-pump arterial pressures < -250 mm Hg indicate the inability of the catheter to deliver the prescribed blood flow (Q_b) and may be indicative of catheter malfunction. With a pre-pump pressure of 180 to 220 mm Hg, roller pump blood flow readings overestimate blood flow by approximately 10 %[7].

- In most cases, early malfunction of the catheter is due to technical problems (e.g. kinking), incorrect placement or secondary dislocation of the catheter tip, which should be placed in the right atrium or at its junction with the superior vena cava. Late dislocation may also occur.
- Clotting of the catheter decreases blood flow and endangers adequacy of dialysis if treatment time is not adjusted, or stops blood flow.
- Catheter infection is common with an incidence of catheter-related bacteraemia of approximately 3.4-5.5/1000 patient days[8, 9, 10]. Catheter care must be performed using aseptic technique (see algorithm "Placement and routine management of permanent Tunneled catheters"). Signs of potential infection are erythema, discharge and pain around the catheter tract with increased WBC or fever. Infection should be evaluated and treated promptly (see Algorithm "Management of Tunneled Catheter Infection").

References see p. 128

Assessment for access placement

Clinical Evaluation of Access Site

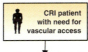
CRI patient with need for vascular access

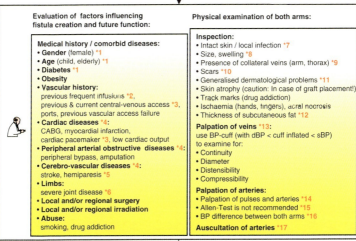

Evaluation of factors influencing fistula creation and future function:

Medical history / comorbid diseases:
- **Gender** (female) *1
- **Age** (child, elderly) *1
- **Diabetes** *1
- **Obesity**
- **Vascular history:**
  previous frequent infusions *2,
  previous & current central-venous access *3,
  ports, previous vascular access failure
- **Cardiac diseases** *4:
  CABG, myocardial infarction,
  cardiac pacemaker *3, low cardiac output
- **Peripheral arterial obstructive diseases** *4:
  peripheral bypass, amputation
- **Cerebro-vascular diseases** *4:
  stroke, hemiparesis *5
- **Limbs:**
  severe joint disease *6
- **Local and/or regional surgery**
- **Local and/or regional irradiation**
- **Abuse:**
  smoking, drug addiction

Physical examination of both arms:

Inspection:
- Intact skin / local infection *7
- Size, swelling *8
- Presence of collateral veins (arm, thorax) *9
- Scars *10
- Generalised dermatological problems *11
- Skin atrophy (caution: In case of graft placement!)
- Track marks (drug addiction)
- Ischaemia (hands, fingers), acral necrosis
- Thickness of subcutaneous fat *12

Palpation of veins *13:
use BP-cuff (with dBP < cuff inflated < sBP)
to examine for:
- Continuity
- Diameter
- Distensibility
- Compressibility

Palpation of arteries:
- Palpation of pulses and arteries *14
- Allen-Test is not recommended *15
- BP difference between both arms *16

Auscultation of arteries *17

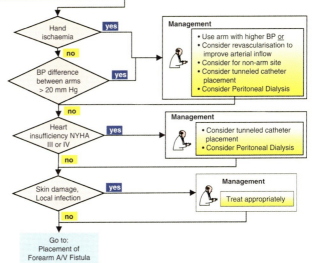

Clinical Evaluation of Access Site

*1 Medical history/concomitant diseases
- Medical history and concomitant diseases have a strong impact on the choice of possible access sites. Vascular access as a matter of principle should be created as distally as possible in order to preserve proximal sites for later.
- Female gender and old age as risk factors influencing fistula creation remain controversial. Elderly and diabetic patients have reduced quality of vessels needed for successful access creation[1]. In diabetic patients, some authors therefore recommend elbow A/V fistulas instead of wrist fistulas[2, 3]. This policy is reasonable in patients with reduced life expectancy irrespective of underlying diagnosis, in whom a single successful access procedure may suffice for the rest of their lives. In younger patients with reasonable life expectancy but with sub-optimal veins and arteries, however, every effort should be made to create a peripheral A/V fistula at the wrist or at the forearm, accepting the increased risk of surgical revision or radiological intervention later.
- Diabetic patients often display medial calcification of their peripheral arteries (especially radial and ulnar arteries). Medial calcification will hinder the maturation process of the A/V fistula by preventing the natural dilatation of the feeding artery and the subsequent increase in arterial flow. Preoperative X-ray of the hand can be performed to look for medial sclerosis. When severe medial sclerosis is present some surgeons avoid radiocephalic A/V fistula creation in favour of an elbow A/V fistula[4]. However, functional distal A/V fistulas have been reported in the presence of calcification although there is a higher risk of failure[5]. The decision of access site has to be made by an experienced access surgeon on an individual basis in each diabetic patient.
- Access surgery is also difficult in small women, children, elderly or obese patients, in patients with breast and oto-rhino-laryngeal cancers, after solid organ transplantation and long-term steroid therapy, due to size, location and damage of vessels. Venography and ultrasonography are of great value in localising suitable veins in such patients[6].
- Cardiac surgery, or clavicular fracture increases the risk for central venous stenosis or occlusion.

*2 Previous venous cannulation
- Venous system cannulation, i.v. drug abuse, intensive intravenous therapy and numerous venous blood sampling often destroy the superficial venous system and in such patients, radiological and ultrasonographic examination has to be done carefully to find a suitable vein for access creation.

*3 Previous and current central venous catheters
- Central venous catheterisation for dialysis, placement of a pacemaker[7] or port for chemotherapy, may cause central venous stenosis or thrombosis, often indicated by clinically obvious venous collateralisation over the shoulder and chest. Thus, creation of an A/V fistula in the upper limb may be impaired, since venous stenosis will become symptomatic once there is increased venous blood flow from the fistula. This condition usually results in a painful swelling of the whole arm[8].

*4 Cardiac / Vascular diseases
- Myocardial infarction, coronary artery bypass grafts, peripheral bypass, stroke or amputation suggest generalised arterial disease. Thus careful clinical, ultrasono-

graphic, and angiographic investigation is mandatory, particularly to assess the quality of the arterial tree[6, 9, 10].
- As stated by Sidawy et al. "contrast arteriography remains the gold standard for the evaluation of a suspected inflow stenosis or occlusion. When in doubt regarding the adequacy of the donor artery or the runoff, it is advisable to obtain an arteriogram that shows the entire arterial system from the origin of the subclavian to the distal branches. Magnetic resonance angiography can also be used for the same purpose"[11].

*5 Stroke and other neurological diseases
- Hemiparesis is thought to cause reduced arterial and venous blood flow rates due to immobility. In most of these patients, the paralysed arm is selected for access creation despite comparatively less suitable vessels in the other upper limb, because the other arm may be used to support walking with crutches and thus the access vein might be exposed to external compression and damage.
- In addition, in selecting the paralysed arm, the healthy arm can be used during the period of haemodialysis, and particularly for puncture site compression after completion of dialysis.
- In a severely disabled limb, however, access creation and cannulation may be difficult or even impossible if severe contracture occurs.

*6 Severe joint disease or vasculitis
- Patients suffering from severe joint disease and vasculitis have often undergone long-term steroid therapy, which often results in vascular complications such as increased arterial wall thickness, arterial stiffness and loss of distensibility. Steroid-induced skin atrophy and immunosuppression enhance the risk for postoperative infectious complications.

*7 Local infection
- Vascular access should be placed only after resolution of local or systemic infection.

*8 Arm swelling
- Inadequate venous drainage may be indicated by swelling of one arm compared to the other, and prominent collateral veins around the shoulder. Such signs are indications for venography. If the underlying anatomic defect cannot be corrected, the limb must not be used for access creation, as an already symptomatic stenosis will become even more so[8].
- In cases of bilateral obstruction, the central venous stenosis or occlusion may be treated by angioplasty or surgical bypass, which should be performed simultaneously to or soon after creation of the A/V fistula. Long-term success is poor.

*9 Presence of collateral veins
- Special attention has to be paid to venous collaterals of the upper arm and shoulder suggesting central venous stenosis.
- The finding of venous collaterals is an indication for bilateral imaging by MRA or venography, using CO_2 or gadolinium in cases of iodine sensitivity.
- Depending on the character of the venous narrowing, an A/V fistula can, nevertheless, be created in some of these patients. With a functioning A/V fistula, interventional procedures such as angioplasty and/or stent insertion can be done much more proficiently and successfully. In some of these patients venous

hypertension after creation of the A/V access will be so mild that a "wait and see" policy may be instituted. Such decisions should be based on the investigator's experience and tailored to the individual patient.

*10 Scars
- Scars in the arm or neck will reveal previous operations, traumatic events and central venous catheterisations. A combination of typical scars and inflammatory signs may be found in a drug addict.

*11 Generalised dermatological problems
- In most patients with generalised dermatological problems, a vascular access can be created using supportive anti-inflammatory therapy recommended by dermatologists.

*12 Thickness of subcutaneous fat
- Obesity can prevent effective palpation of the forearm and upper arm veins. On the other hand, an absent subcutaneous fatty layer may increase the risk of skin necrosis, especially when the insertion of graft material is necessary.
- Subcutaneous fat usually preserves superficial veins from venipuncture and cannulation. These veins are often of very good quality but frequently will necessitate transposition into a more superficial location after fistula creation.

*13 Palpation of veins
- Examination should take place in a warm room. A tourniquet should be placed around the upper arm or a blood pressure cuff inflated to 40 mm Hg in order to produce sufficient venous distension. For examination of the proximal upper arm veins a band tourniquet close to the axilla can be used. The anatomical course of the forearm cephalic and basilic veins should then be inspected and palpated. The veins should be distensible (up to 2-3 mm), patent and without stenosis up to the elbow in order to provide a good A/V fistula. By light percussion of the vein at the wrist, a transmitted pulse wave should be felt in the vein at the elbow and vice versa, proving the patency of the vein.
- In addition to the forearm veins, the great veins of the upper arm should be evaluated carefully. By exerting different pressures with a blood pressure cuff, diameter, continuity, distensibility and compressibility of the veins are controlled. In venous thrombosis, these characteristic clinical signs are usually absent.
- Venous imaging by either colour-coded duplex-ultrasound, venography or MRI is indicated when no vein clinically appears to be usable in both forearms. Venography or MRI should be performed, when a central venous obstruction is suspected (see **derma*8** and **derma*9**).

*14 Palpation of arterial pulses
- Palpation characterises the pulses of the brachial, radial and ulnar artery, giving initial information on the quality of the arterial tree. The pulse of the brachial artery is palpated at the medial side of the elbow, the radial pulse 2 cm proximal of the proc. stylodius radii and the ulnar pulse 2 cm proximal of the proc. styloidius ulnae, to check for any obvious signs of calcification and atherosclerosis impairing the arterial inflow. The pulses are graded as "normal", "diminished" and "absent"[11] and compared with the contralateral limb.

*15 The Allen-Test
- The Allen test is a very subjective assessment of distal hand circulation with

variable outcome. Its value in the assessment for A/V fistula placement remains controversial and of limited value (see appendix for details).

*16 Blood pressure difference
- Systolic and diastolic blood pressures should be measured in both arms according to the Riva-Rocci method, in the supine position. An index of the systolic blood pressure of the ipsilateral arm with the systolic blood pressure of the contralateral arm is calculated:

$$\text{AAI (arm/arm index)} = \frac{\text{systolic blood pressure projected fistula arm}}{\text{systolic blood pressure contralateral arm}}$$

- Significant proximal arterial disease is likely with an AAI < 0.90. There should be a blood pressure difference of less than 20 mm Hg in the upper limb selected for A/V fistula creation, compared to the contralateral limb. For creating an A/V fistula, a difference in blood pressure below 20 mm Hg is chosen as an non invasive criterion for the selection of upper extremity arterias[12].

*17 Auscultation of arteries
- In presence of an arterial stenosis, auscultation along the axillary and subclavian artery can reveal a high-frequency bruit.
- More detailed information on the quality of the arterial system is provided by duplex scanning[6], which is highly recommended and is evidence based.

References see p. 129

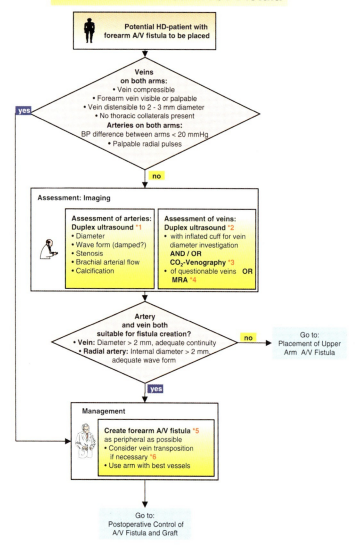

Placement of Forearm A/V Fistula

Despite the increasing number of patients with diabetes, peripheral vascular disease and of older age, creation of a native A/V fistula is possible in the vast majority of cases[1, 2]. Konner et al. created 748 primary A/V fistulas – but only 52 % were located in the forearm – in patients, of whom 24 % had diabetes as their cause of end stage renal disease, without the use of graft material[3]. One year primary access survival ranged from 70 % (in male patients with diabetes mellitus and under the age of 65) to 85 % (male, non-DM, < 65 years), secondary access survival was 84 % (male, DM, < 65 years) to 98 % (male, non-DM, < 65 years).

The early occlusion or failure of the fistula vein to dilate rate, as reported in the literature from 1983 to 1986, were higher, ranging from 10 to 24 %[4, 5, 6, 7, 8, 9] and the success rates of early revisions were often less than 50 %. This high failure rate may be primarily due to the selection of inappropriate vessels or due to stenosis at the anastomosis, impairing adequate blood flow. Lower early failure rates of 5.6 % and 8.3 % were reported by Mihmanli et al. in 2001 and by Silva et al. in 1998, respectively[10, 11] but is likely to reflect a very selective policy. In order to select the most appropriate vessels for the creation of the native A/V fistulas, many authors recommend the use of duplex-ultrasound investigation before each fistula creation[12, 10, 11, 13, 14, 15, 16].

It is difficult to compare failure rates, as there are two different "schools of thinking". Some teams attempt fistula creation only when the arteries and veins are of optimal quality. If these conditions are not found at the wrist, the A/V fistula is created at the elbow or the upper arm. One significant concern is that if the radiocephalic fistula occludes then there is a risk that the radial artery may also occlude. Steal syndrome may be more likely to occur when an elbow fistula is created later in the same arm, especially in a diabetic patient. In contrast other surgeons, especially those using microsurgery and working in close cooperation with interventional radiologists, will attempt fistula creation even when venography or duplex shows evidence of small but non-stenosed vessels. The latter bears the risk of higher initial failure rates and delay in achieving a functional vascular access for the patient but less risk of mid-term and long-term morbidity and mortality since steal syndromes and excessive high flows are much less frequent in forearm fistulas. Two recently published articles stress the value of interventional radiology in helping failing fistulas to mature[17, 18].

*1 Assessment of arteries: Duplex ultrasound

- Duplex ultrasound (see appendix) is an accurate method for the investigation of arteries in the upper extremity with a sensitivity of 90 % and a specificity of 99 % for the detection of obstructive disease and is strongly recommended, pre- and post operatively, for the assessment of vessels and fistula outcome[19]. The use of duplex ultrasound influences the choice of access placement[13].
- Vessel diameter measured by duplex ultrasound can be potentially underestimated, as the vessel might be in spasm or insufficiently distended during the investigation. The procedure should be performed in a warm room to reduce the risk of vasospasm. In cases of severe calcification, it can be impossible to measure the diameter of the artery.
- A standardised examination is performed starting from the infraclavicular subclavian artery down to the brachial, radial and ulnar arteries at the wrist. Arterial diameters, Doppler waveform analysis and sites of stenosis or occlusion are

recorded. Adequate arterial inflow is of prime importance for successful functioning of A/V fistulas.
- Duplex ultrasonography was used in one study to determine the change in resistance index (RI) at reactive hyperaemia as a test of the functional status of the feeding artery (see appendix 1.2.6 for details). A/V fistulas were successfully created in 95.3 % cases when using feeding arteries with a RI at reactive hyperaemia of < 0.7 and only 38.7 % with an RI of > .
- The internal radial artery diameter has been used in several studies to predict the outcome of radiocephalic (RC) A/V fistulas (failure or dysmaturation) or to plan strategies for vascular access creation. Wong et al. observed either thrombosis or failure to maturation in all RC A/V fistulas created in patients with either a radial artery or a cephalic vein with a diameter < 1.6 mm[21]. In another study, successful A/V fistulas had a preoperatively measured radial artery diameter of 2.7 mm versus 1.9 mm in failed A/V fistulas[14]. Malovrh discriminated between RC A/V fistula created with radial arteries, whose diameter were > 1.5 mm versus ≤ 1.5 mm. Immediate patency rate in the >1.5 mm group was 92 % versus 45 % in the ≤ 1.5 mm group, while the patency rates after 12 weeks were 83 % versus 36 %, respectively[12]. However it has to be stressed that lower success rates with smaller vessels do not necessarily mean that A/V fistula creation must not be attempted.
- In the study performed by Silva et al. strategy for vascular access creation was based on preoperative duplex scanning. Patients with a radial artery diameter of ≥ 2 mm and a cephalic vein of ≥ 2.5 mm received RC A/V fistulas, while grafts were used in patients with insufficient radial arteries and cephalic veins and an outflow vein in the elbow with a diameter of ≥ 4 mm. The percentage of RC A/V fistula creation increased from 14 % to 63 %, while the early failure rate decreased from 36 % to 8 %[11]. The percentage of A/V fistulas in this study could have been higher, if antecubital veins of 4 mm or more had been used to create an autogenous fistula at the elbow.

Table 1 summarises the findings of several authors on minimal arterial diameters necessary for successful creation of radiocephalic A/V fistulas. These are still debatable and controversial as cut-off points for A/V fistula creation. The lack of consensus also indicates that vessel diameter alone is insufficient to guarantee fistula success as pointed out by Wong et al.

Table 1:
Minimum radial artery diameter for successful creation of radiocephalic A/V fistulas in adults:

Author	*Radial artery diameter*
Wong et al.[21]	1.6 mm
Silva et al.[11]	2.0 mm
Malovrh et al.[12]	1.5 mm

Soft tissues X-rays
- A simple film of the forearms can show calcifications of the forearm arteries, which

does not contraindicate fistula creation but may warn the surgeon of potential difficulties. Palpation of the artery is usually sufficient, however.

Digital angiography or MRA
- Contrast arteriography remains the gold standard for the evaluation of a suspected arterial stenosis or occlusion. When results of clinical examination and colour-coded duplex-ultrasound are suggestive of arterial run-in or run-off problems, it is advisable to obtain an arteriogram that shows the entire arterial system from the origin of the subclavian artery to the distal forearm branches. Magnetic resonance angiography can also be used for the same purpose[22].

*2 Assessment of veins: Duplex ultrasound
- The veins in the upper extremity are investigated in the supine position with a tourniquet placed on the forearm, and subsequently moved to the upper arm. The cephalic and basilic veins at the wrist are assessed for compressibility and diameter. Furthermore, the forearm veins are followed proximally for continuity and size. At the antecubital fossa, vein continuity and diameters are verified. After removal of the tourniquet, the continuity of the deep system is determined through the axillary and subclavian veins. The predictive value of cephalic vein diameters for successful RC A/V fistulas remains uncertain. Vein diameters of < 1.6 mm have been associated with A/V fistula failure[21], while good patency rates were obtained in patients with A/V fistulas that were created on the basis of the selection of adequate veins (diameter of the cephalic vein at the wrist ≥ 2-2.5 mm or upper arm veins > 3 mm)[23].
- However, despite the lower success rates with smaller vessels, some groups would still attempt fistula creation. In children microsurgery allows for the successful use of even smaller veins and arteries[24, 25]. Children's vessels are different form those of adults, however, and have a much better capacity to develop. It has been speculated that a skilful surgical technique, possibly including microsurgery, may also enhance patency rates in adults with marginal vessel quality, although there has been no randomised trial to corroborate this conviction.
- The size of the increase in vein diameter after proximal vein compression before fistula creation could also be an important predictor of success. In a recently published study, in the group of successfully created A/V fistula, the vein diameter increased by 48 %. In contrast, vein diameter only increased by 11.8 % in the group with early failure of the A/V fistula[20].

Table 2 summarises the recommendation on minimum vein diameter:

Table 2:
Minimum cephalic vein diameter for successful creation of radiocephalic A/V fistulas in adults:

Author	Cephalic vein
Wong et al.[21]	1.6 mm
Malovrh et al.[20]	1.6 mm
Silva et al.[11]	2.5 mm
Ascher et al.[23]	2.0 mm

*3 **Venography** (see also appendix)
- Venography of the arm veins with iodine-contrast may cause further deterioration of renal function in the pre-dialysis patient. Therefore, the patient will need adequate hydration with urinary diuresis and as little contrast as possible. Alternatively, CO_2-venography can be used, although it raises other risks and should be performed by experienced radiologists only.
- Gadolinum may also serve as an alternative to jodine as a contrast agent. Rieger et al. performed 32 angiographic procedures (for other reasons than A/V fistula creation) in 29 CRI patients with gadopentetate dimeglumine[26]. In only one patient, serum creatinine concentration increased by more than 0.5 mg/dl after the procedure, although this may have been due to cholesterol embolism as a complication of renal artery stenting, rather than caused by the contrast medium.
- While gadoterate meglumine is regarded as an effective and safe contrast agent for upper extremity venography for the planning of an A/V fistula[27], others argue that Gadolinum is more toxic than iodine at equal attenuating concentrations[28]. Gadolinum is also more expensive than conventional contrast media or CO_2.

*4 **Magnetic resonance angiography (MRA)** (see also appendix)
- Magnetic resonance angiography (MRA), with either time-of-flight (TOF) or contrast-enhanced (Gadolinum) technique, is a promising new diagnostic tool. The latter technique results in a good visualisation of arm veins. Conventional and MRA venographic diameter measurements were closely correlated overall ($r = 0.91$) and on a vein-to-vein basis ($r = 0.84–0.98$)[29]. However, this study has been criticised, since veins were imaged without placement of a tourniquet, which is essential to produce good venous filling and dilatation. In addition, upper arm and central veins were not studied[30].

*5 **Create forearm A/V fistula**
- Forearm fistulas, especially wrist fistulas, show several advantages over upper arm fistulas: They preserve more proximal vessels for future access placement, have lower complication rates such as vascular steal syndrome, thrombosis and infection, better long-term patency rates[31] and a longer vein length for dialysis needling. Such fistulas rarely cause excessive high flow due to dilatation of the feeding artery, even when they remain patent for many years.
- After thrombosis and declotting by interventional radiology, the one-year secondary patency rates in forearm A/V fistulas and upper arm A/V fistulas were 81 % and 50 %, respectively in one study[32].
- An increasing percentage of patients nearing ESRD do not have a forearm vein and a forearm artery suitable for vascular access creation. In these patients, the A/V fistula should be created using the veins and arteries of the middle of the forearm, the region below the elbow or at the elbow region[1]. In summary, in the vast majority of patients with a damaged arterial and venous vascular system, the question is not only to ask for the dominant or non-dominant arm, but to evaluate the best location where an arterio-venous access can be placed successfully. The selection of the left or right arm primarily depends on the quality of the vessels although in principle the non-dominant arm is preferred in order to keep the dominant arm free for the patient to use during dialysis. The selection of the anastomotic site in these problematic cases must not be done based merely on the results of a clinical examination, but only after adequate pre-operative non-invasive or invasive vascular mapping.

- Ligation of venous side branches should be avoided during access creation. The pattern of venous dilatation/arterialisation cannot be foreseen at the time of the first operation. In case of a formerly undetected obstruction of the proximal "main" vein, collateralisation via branches can occasionally provide successful cannulation sites and act as run off to prevent fistula thrombosis
- When the "main" access vein and its collaterals fail to dilate over time, imaging by duplex ultrasound or by angiography must be performed and the underlying stenosis must be then treated by percutaneous dilatation or by creation of a new anastomosis if the stenosis is close to the anastomosis. Sometimes, there are two main veins taking fistula flow and neither may develop sufficiently for dialysis needling. If one of such veins is ligated then the other vein is likely to mature suitable for needling. Otherwise, there is little room if any for ligation or embolisation in correctly performed autogenous A/V fistulas.
- End artery to end vein should be avoided as only in end vein to side artery or in side to side anastomoses, distal arterial flow can contribute to the flow of the A/V fistula, ranging from 0-50 %[7, 20, 33, 34]. As side to side anastomoses are more likely to cause distal venous hypertension due to possible retrograde venous drainage[35-37], end vein to side artery seems to be the most appropriate form of A/V fistula anastomoses.

*6 Consider vein transposition if necessary
- Superficial venous transposition increases the potential to create forearm A/V fistulas. Silva et al. transposed suitable forearm veins which were not in immediate proximity to a suitable artery. The primary cumulative patency rates after one and two years were 84 % and 69 %, respectively[38].
- Venous transposition in a primary access operation in the forearm should be practised with caution. During maturation, the vein undergoes a process of dilatation, elongation and increase in thickness. These factors are not predictable in cases when the vein is largely mobilised, as this causes trauma to the vasa vasorum and removal of the adventitia[39]. Venous transposition is easier and more successfully achieved in revisions using a dilated, elongated and wall-thickened venous segment, as in a two stage brachiobasilic transposed A/V fistula.

References see p. 130

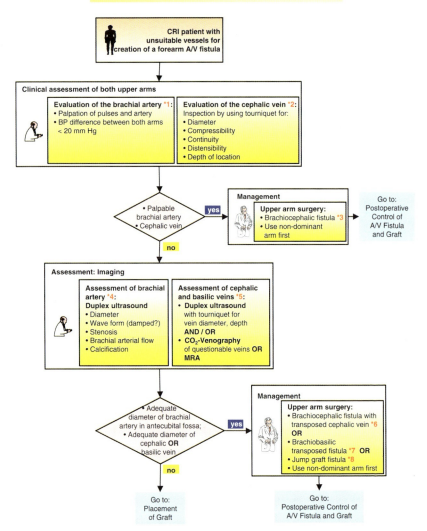

Placement of Elbow or Upper Arm A/V Fistula

Fistulas can also be created in the upper arm or at the elbow. These fistulas are a good alternative, when wrist fistulas cannot be created. Whilst proximal fistulas are recommended by some authors as the first access in patients with diabetes[1, 2], others feel peripheral access can be successfully created. In 2000, Rodriguez reported much better long-term secondary patency rates for forearm fistulas compared with upper arm fistulas (50 % secondary patency at 7 years for forearm fistulas versus 3.6 years for brachiocephalic fistulas and 5 years for brachiobasilic fistulas)[3].

In an article published in 1977, Kinnaert reported 2 years' secondary patency rates ranging from 78.5 % to 100 % for end to side radiocephalic fistulas, and 61 % for ulnar-basilic fistulas. In another article published in 1994, he reported secondary patency rates for upper arm fistulas ranging from 69 % to 80 % at 1 year and from 49 % to 68 % at 4 years [3-5]. Data by Dixon et al.[6] favour upper arm A/V fistulas. The group found higher 1-, 3- and 5-year patency rates in upper arm fistulas (71 %, 57 % and 57 %) compared to forearm A/V fistulas (54 %, 46 % and 36 %) and grafts (54 %, 28 %, 0 %), but upper arm A/V fistulas required more interventions than forearm A/V fistulas (1.0 versus 0.6 per access, respectively).

*1 Evaluation of brachial artery

- Inspection may occasionally reveal a meandering brachial artery, in some cases appearing like a true arterial aneurysm. This is found in patients with other signs of severe atherosclerotic disease, particularly in patients with diabetes mellitus and nephrosclerosis.
- Palpation of the brachial artery along the upper arm should be performed bilaterally to compare the quality of the pulses. A high brachial artery bifurcation occurs in 19 % of patients. In diabetics, however, the artery may be difficult to palpate due to calcification.
- Auscultation revealing a high-frequency bruit along the subclavian / axillary artery in combination with a blood pressure difference exceeding 20 mm Hg may be a sign of impaired arterial supply of the extremity.

*2 Evaluation of cephalic vein

- The cephalic vein lies on the outer side of the upper arm on the medial border of the deltoid muscle. It passes subcutaneously from the elbow upwards and turns subfascially in the upper arm before it joins the subclavian vein. The vein may be visible, but usually can only be palpated. A tourniquet is applied as high as possible in the axilla and the vein is then examined by palpation along its course. Size, compressibility and patency are judged. If the vein cannot be felt because of its deep position, additional imaging techniques like colour Doppler ultrasound may be necessary[7].

*3 Brachiocephalic fistula

- The brachiocephalic A/V fistula is only one of a great variety of possible A/V anastomoses in the elbow region. The individual topography of veins and arteries determines the type of fistula chosen. Depending on the individual situation, the proximal radial artery, the distal brachial artery just above its bifurcation or even the proximal ulnar artery can be used to create the A/V anastomosis. The final determinant for the choice of artery is its diameter and the quality of its wall. The arte-

rial wall should ideally be without calcification. As for forearm fistulas, the brachiocephalic fistula should provide an optimal position for cannulation.
- Brachiocephalic fistulas can be created by an end-cephalic vein to side-brachial artery anastomosis at the elbow. A second possibility is to form an anastomosis between the perforating vein of the median cubital vein and the brachial artery, called the Gracz A/V fistula (for details: see appendix).
- The complication rate is less than in grafts[8], but such fistulas may cause high-output cardiac failure in the long-term[9] or steal phenomena in the short-term[10]. Patency and complication rates of standard brachiocephalic and the Gracz type A/V fistulas are similar[5, 11].

*4 Assessment of brachial artery by duplex ultrasound
- A standardised duplex ultrasound (see appendix) examination of the brachial artery in the supine patient should be performed. Brachial artery diameter, Doppler waveform, flow measurement and vessel wall characteristics are evaluated. Normal diameters of brachial arteries range from 2.5 to 4 mm. With adequate arterial inflow a typical tri-phasic Doppler waveform with a rapid systolic upslope, reversed flow and low diastolic flow is anticipated. Stenosis in the artery results in flattening of the systolic peak with absence of reversed flow. Vessel wall calcification may be noticed by echolucent shadows. An arterial inflow of ≥ 40 ml/min is associated with better outcome of the A/V fistula[12].

*5 Assessment of cephalic and basilic veins
- A standardised duplex ultrasound (see appendix) examination of the cephalic vein from the elbow up to its junction with the subclavian vein and also of the basilic vein at the medial side of the elbow up to its junction with the deep axillary veins should be performed if the clinical examination does not completely clarify the anatomical situation. Vein diameters, compressibility and continuity are checked with a tourniquet placed as high as possible in the axilla. In particular, the location of the junction of the basilic and deep veins is recorded. Because of its deep location duplex investigation of the basilic vein is recommended, although the anatomic position does protect it from cannulation. A diameter of 3-4 mm is desirable for the creation of a brachiocephalic or brachiobasilic A/V fistula[13], however, the continuity and the absence of stenosis are more important than the absolute diameter of the vein.
- (For comments on CO_2 venography and MRA see *2 Placement of Forearm A/V Fistula.)

*6 Brachiocephalic fistula with transposed cephalic vein
- Normally, the cephalic vein is in an ideal subcutaneous position and cannulation can usually be performed successfully. The subcutaneous transposition of the cephalic vein may be necessary only in very obese patients. The fatty tissue layer can often simply be resected resulting in a subcutaneous position of the cephalic vein thus allowing for easy cannulation. Transposition of the vein into a new subcutaneous tunnel apart from the incision needed for mobilisation of the vein, however, is preferred by some groups, because the vein then does not lie beneath scar tissue.

*7 Brachiobasilic transposed fistula
- First described by Dagher et al. in 1976[14] the brachiobasilic anastomosis with con-

secutive mobilisation of the arterialised vein into a subcutaneous position[5] is still superior to the insertion of a graft.
- Rivers et al. investigated the patency rate in brachiobasilic transposed A/V fistulas. After 30 months, 49 % of fistulas were patent[15]. In a pilot study, Hibberd described a patency rate of 70 % after one year in brachiobasilic fistula, while Burkhard and Cikrit found a patency rate of 90 % after one year[16, 17]. Infection and thrombosis occur less often than in grafts, and though they are more likely to mature than brachiocephalic fistulas, they are more susceptible to late thrombosis[18, 19]. On the other hand, Rodrigues et al. found better secondary patency rates in brachiobasilic fistulas when compared to brachiocephalic fistulas[3]. In summary, there is no doubt that the technique of subcutaneous placement of an arterialised basilic vein is superior to graft insertion. However, there has been no clinical trial comparing these two types of upper arm A/V fistulas, so no definitive advice can be given. Selection of the appropriate A/V fistula will depend on quality and topography of the vessels involved.

*8 **Jump graft fistula**
- It is also possible to create a jump graft fistula, using a short interposition graft with a diameter of 6 mm between the brachial artery and the cephalic vein when the latter is diseased or occluded at the elbow level[20]. However, this operation actually changes the autogenous fistula partially into a graft, with all the well-known potential drawbacks of grafts at the venous anastomosis. The alternative is to fully mobilise the cephalic vein and anastomose to a more proximal site on the brachial artery.

References see p. 133

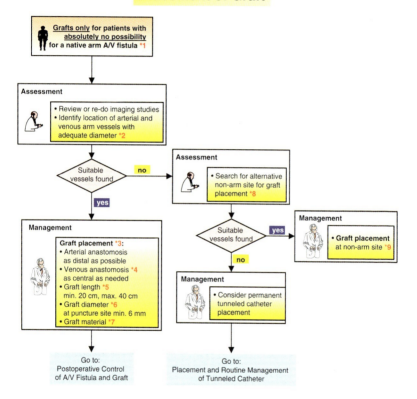

Placement of Graft

*1 Grafts only for patients with no possibility of an autogenous arm A/V fistula
- In general, native A/V fistulas must always be preferred to grafts, as grafts are associated with higher rates of infection[1, 2, 3] and thrombosis[1, 4]. Even after successful thrombolysis of thrombosed grafts, the outcome in grafts is worse than in autogenous A/V fistulas[5] thus leading to high rates of intervention and revision[1, 6, 7]. Thrombosis occurs at a rate of 0.5 – 2.5 events/patient year[8] compared to 0.2 events per patient year in native A/V fistulas. Failure rates are 20 % and 10 % per year for grafts and native A/V fistulas, respectively (see appendix III for details).
- In addition, the mortality risks in patients with grafts and especially with central venous catheters is increased when compared to patients with native A/V fistulas[9].
- For those patients who start dialysis with a central venous catheter and who then develop life-threatening catheter-related morbidity, the lead time needed to perform, await development of or create a secondary access if the first one fails, may result in an unacceptably high risk. In such **exceptional** patients, a peripheral arteriovenous graft may serve as an alternative to an arteriovenous fistula, despite the poorer long-term result with grafts. This provision does not condone graft insertion except in very exceptional cases.
- In elderly patients not suitable for autogenous proximal access, a proximal brachioaxillary prosthetic graft is considered a good alternative[10]. Grafts have a low early failure rate of < 6 % (see appendix III), but face the risk of thrombotic occlusion due to impairment of flow caused by intimal hyperplasia-related stenoses at the venous anastomosis. Without a surveillance program and active interventional treatment of stenotic lesions, the patency rate of grafts is rather low with 29-60 % at 1 year[11, 12] and approximately 40 % after 2 years[11]. With surveillance and intervention with percutaneous transluminal angioplasty (PTA), the thrombosis rate can be reduced to less than 0.5 thromboses / patient-year[8].

*2 Identify location of arterial and venous arm vessels with adequate diameter
- An objective assessment of arm arteries and veins is obligatory especially if a lack of suitable vessels for primary radiocephalic A/V fistulas is suspected or if previous A/V fistulas have failed. A standardised duplex scan is performed with special emphasis on elbow and upper arm basilic/cephalic/antecubital veins and deep veins. Also, the diameter and the quality of axillary and brachial artery are examined. An outflow vein of > 3.5 – 4 mm is thought most appropriate for graft implantation[13, 11], although there is no prospective study proving this.

*3 Graft Placement
- Haemodialysis access grafts should be implanted only after exhaustion of superficial veins in both upper extremities.
- Forearm straight grafts (from distal radial artery to antecubital or peripheral brachial vein) provide a sufficient graft length (20 cm or more) in normal sized adults. However, if a suitable vein for graft placement is found in the elbow, this vein might also be suitable for the creation of a native A/V fistula.
- Upper arm grafts should be sutured to the larger veins found in the upper third of the arm. The first graft-to-vein anastomosis should not be performed high in the axilla, since surgical revision of anastomotic stenosis is easier and can be performed under local anaesthesia.

- Different outcomes have been described in looped compared to straight grafts. Lazarides et al. described a higher risk of access failure in straight forearm grafts compared to looped forearm grafts, from antecubital artery to antecubital or peripheral brachial vein. However, there is a risk of steal syndrome when the graft is placed on the brachial artery but not when placed on the radial artery. In the upper arm, looped grafts performed worse than straight grafts, from distal brachial artery to axillary vein[14]. The better patency rates of looped grafts in the forearm may be due to the larger diameter of the artery at the anastomosis and/or due to the haemodynamically favourable antegrade inflow. However, forearm grafts can preclude later creation of an elbow fistula. Upper arm grafts should be performed only after failure of forearm and elbow fistulas (transposed brachiobasilic fistulas included)[14].
- When the subclavian vein is occluded, brachial artery to jugular vein grafts or axillary artery-to-internal jugular vein cross-over grafts should be considered (see Algorithm "Management of Central Venous Stenosis (2)", ***7**)[15, 16, 17, 18]. Patency and complication rates are comparable to those of upper arm grafts, although the number of such procedures is small.
- Graft placement can be performed largely as an outpatient procedure[19], thus reducing costs, although the age and infirmity of the patient needs to be taken into account, and not cost alone.

*4 Venous anastomosis
- For reasons of preservation of the venous tree, the venous graft anastomosis should be placed as peripherally as possible. Veins below the antecubital fossa, however, do not usually have a diameter of 4 mm or more needed to guarantee graft patency[11]. Therefore, forearm grafts will end at the antecubital fossa or even above the elbow.
- While it is obvious that the arterial graft anastomosis is to be sutured in an end graft to side artery fashion, comparative studies on venous end-to-side versus end-to-end anastomosis are absent. A vein cuff to widen the venous end-to-side anastomosis has not been shown to improve patency rates[11]. Early graft failure is correlated with the initial diameter of the vein at the anastomosis. Suturing the graft to a vein smaller than 4 mm is not ideal[11].
- A graft usually will not sustain a blood pressure < 100 mm Hg, so it should not be placed into a haemodynamically unstable patient.

*5 Graft length
- The length of the graft should exceed 20 cm to provide at least 15 cm for rope-ladder puncture with two needles. Excessive graft length (> 40 cm) is believed to be associated with higher thrombosis rates.

*6 Graft diameter
- The ideal graft diameter still remains to be defined. Small calibre grafts, make needling difficult, whereas large diameter grafts run the risk of high arterio-venous flow with consequent cardiac stress and/or peripheral steal syndrome. Therefore, 6 mm or 7 mm grafts are a widely accepted compromise.
- In order to reduce midgraft stenosis observed with smaller graft sizes, Polo et al. tapered an 8 mm graft to 6 mm at the arterial anastomosis. Primary and secondary patency rates at 1, 3 and 5 years were 73 %, 53 %, 41 % and 91 %, 80 % and 72 %, respectively[20]. In a second study, Polo et al. compared primary and sec-

ondary patency rates in grafts of 6 mm and 6-8 mm. Primary patency rates were 62 %, 58 % and 44 % in 6 mm grafts and 85 %, 78 %, and 73 % in 6-8 mm grafts at year 1, 2 and 3. Secondary patency rates remained stable during the first three years at 85 % for 6 mm and 90 % for 6-8 mm grafts, respectively (unpublished data).

*7 **Graft material**
- Expanded polytetrafluoroethylene (ePTFE) is the most frequently used graft material for prosthetic vascular access and recommended by the K/DOQI guidelines[21]. In clinical trials ePTFE has been compared to other graft materials such as plasma tetrafluoroethylene[21, 22], or polyurethane[23]. In these studies, none of the alternatives performed better than ePTFE. Standard wall thickness ePTFE provides better patency rates than thin-walled ePTFE[24] (see Appendix III for details).
- Tordoir et al. found higher patency rates in stretch ePTFE grafts than in standard ePTFE gratts[12].
- PTFE grafts have a high incidence of postoperative infection which is 6 % during the initial 30 days. Zibari et al. were able to reduce the incidence of infection down to 1 % with 750 mg of vancomycin i.v. given 6-12 hours before the operation[25]. Others feel that this policy may induce resistance to this important antibiotic and prefer to use a cephalosporin. However, there has been no randomised controlled trial. With a preoperative dose of 2 grams of Cephalzoline, 30 days infection rates can also be as low as 0.9 %[26].

*8 **Non-arm sites for graft placement**
- Only in those rare cases when the arterial and venous trees of both arms (including the axillary arteries and veins) are unsuitable for arterio-venous access, non-arm sites should be considered. Basically, a bridge graft can connect virtually any artery to any vein to form an arterio-venous access. Artery and vein should preferably have a diameter exceeding 4 mm[11], and the veins central to the graft have to be free from obstruction. Colour-coded duplex ultrasound is the method of choice to define the vessels best suitable. In questionable cases, angiography and/or venography need to be performed.

*9 **Graft placement at non-arm site**
- The thigh is the next common site for fistula creation after the upper limbs.
- Several options exist for autogenous AV fistulas in the thigh, such as transposition of the long saphenous vein (if not already translocated to the arm to create an AV fistula) or superficial femoral vein (SFV). Gradman et al. constructed AV fistulas using the transposed SFV, with primary and secondary patency at one year of 73 % and 86 % respectively[28]. No infection occurred and 7 patients required PTFE graft insertion.
- The PTFE graft fistula is the commonest type of vascular access created in the thigh. Patency and complication rates of lower limb grafts are comparable to those of upper arm grafts[27]. A straight graft can be anastomosed to the popliteal artery or distal superficial femoral artery and Tunneled up to the long saphenous vein or common femoral vein in the groin, or, in reverse, from a femoral artery down to the origin of the superficial femoral vein in the distal thigh. Alternatively a femoro-femoral looped graft can be performed. The arterial in-flow can be from all three groin arteries – the common femoral artery, profunda femoris or the superficial femoral artery (SFA) origin. The advantage of the profunda or superficial femoral

artery is that in the rare instance when there is serious infection of the graft arterial anastomosis, the profunda or SFA can be ligated without compromising perfusion of the whole leg, as would happen in ligating the common femoral artery.
- The femoral artery-to-femoral vein looped bridge graft is the most frequently performed fistula in the lower limb.

References see p. 134

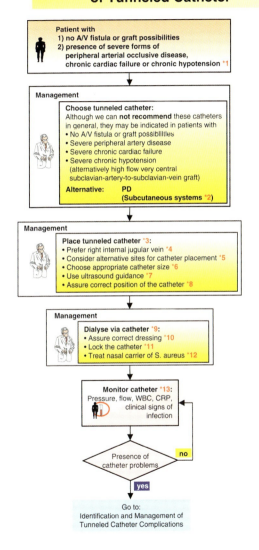

Placement and Routine Management of Tunneled Catheter

*1 **Patients with severe peripheral arterial obstructive disease, chronic cardiac failure, or chronic hypotension**
- Central venous catheters for dialysis are necessary in patients in whom adequate access blood flow cannot be sustained without steal syndrome or deleterious effects on the general circulation.

*2 **Subcutaneous devices**
- Although some papers indicate that infectious complications might also be reduced by subcutaneously implantable port-systems[1], data in the literature does not suggest that infection rates are lower in ports than in Tunneled catheters.
- In addition, these systems may suffer from mechanical complications (see Appendix III) and are also expensive.

*3 **Place permanent tunneled catheter**
- Permanent central venous catheters should only be placed by trained and experienced staff. The procedure should be performed in a dedicated clean area under aseptic conditions[2]. Surgical asepsis includes hand washing at least for two minutes, sterile gloves, facial mask, and an assistant required to support the procedure.

*4 **Preference for the right internal jugular vein**
- The right internal jugular vein is preferred for catheter placement due to its direct continuity into the superior vena cava and the right atrium[3], and catheter length is shorter.
- In acute catheters, blood flow rates achieved in the left internal jugular vein were lower than those obtained in the right internal jugular vein[4].
- A left internal jugular catheter can also produce left brachiocephalic vein stenosis and occlusion
- If an A/V fistula or graft is planned to be used in the future, the cuffed catheter should be placed in the internal jugular vein contralateral to the planned or developing A/V fistula or PTFE graft.
- Thrombosis of the central vein after catheter insertion is a serious problem. Catheter placement in the subclavian vein must be avoided[3] due to higher complication rates and a higher incidence of developing central vein stenosis (42 – 50 % with subclavian vein catheters vs. 0 – 10 % with internal jugular vein catheters)[5, 6] or thrombosis (13 % with subclavian vein catheters vs. 3 % with internal jugular vein catheters)[7].
- Central vein stenosis often remains asymptomatic until creation of an ipsilateral arteriovenous access. G. Jean investigated 51 patients by upper limb phlebography while or after being dialysed on internal jugular vein tunneled CVC during a mean period of 28 months. 24 patients (47 %) had one or more central vein, from the subclavian vein to the superior and the inferior vena cava, high grade stenosis > 50 %, or complete occlusion. 5 of the 12 patients with subclavian vein stenosis had never had any subclavian catheter[8].

*5 **Consider alternative sites for catheter placement**
- Other potential catheter placement sites include the femoral vein, inferior vena cava through a translumbar approach and transhepatic placement. Femoral catheters have been reported to require more interventions and to cause more

infections than thoracic ones[9]. In a prospective study 80 % of femoral catheters required anticoagulation compared to 16 % of jugular catheters[10]. Nevertheless a median survival of tunneled femoral catheters of 166 days was reported[11].

*6 Choose appropriate catheter size

- Catheters used should be designed to provide blood flow rates > 350 ml/min[12]. Catheters with a size of 10 to 12 French generally allow a blood flow up to 250 ml/min[13], as the main determinant of flow is the diameter of the catheter (Poiseuille's Law)[14].
- Longer catheters provide less blood flow at the same inflow pressure compared to shorter catheters of the same diameter. Consequently, in larger patients, where longer catheters are used, the blood flow rate may be lower than in smaller patients, making it more difficult to administer the appropriate dialysis dose[15].
- When the femoral vein is used for haemodialysis access, the length of the catheter must be 20 cm or more, and the catheter tip should at least be positioned in the common iliac vein although preferably in the inferior vena cava. With the tip of a shorter catheter positioned in the external iliac vein, high rates of recirculation will be encountered[16, 17].

*7 Use ultrasound guidance

- Due to the anatomic variability of the venous system and the high rate of complications (5.9 %) including pneumo- and haemothorax, arterial puncture, air embolism, atrial perforation, recurrent laryngeal nerve palsy and cardiac arrest[13], real-time ultrasonic guidance is strongly recommended[15].
- In internal jugular vein catheters, the use of ultrasound-guidance increases the rate of successful placement (100 % with compared to 88.1 % without ultrasound guidance)[18] and decreases the rate of complications including haematoma and carotid artery puncture[18, 19, 20].
- Kwon et al. compared cannulation of the femoral vein with ultrasound guidance to the cannulation by the landmark technique. They described a 100 % success rate in 28 patients using the ultrasound guidance compared to 89.5 % success in 38 patients using the landmark technique[21].

*8 Assure correct position of the catheter

- Blood flow, which should reach > 300 ml/min, depends on the catheter tip location, the status of the patient's central circulation[13] and the catheter design. The catheter tip should be positioned in the mid right atrium to allow adequate flow[22, 23].
- Be aware of the retraction of the catheter tip by as much as 1 to 2 cm, when the patient adopts an upright position, as the chest wall is pulled downward[3], particularly in obese patients or women with large breasts.
- Advancing the catheter into the lower atrium must be avoided, as this may cause dysrhythmias[3].

*9 Dialysis via catheter

- In order to minimise the risk of infection the catheter should only be used for dialysis[2].
- Only trained dialysis staff should perform catheter connection, disconnection and interventions under aseptic conditions. The patient and staff member should wear a surgical mask[2].

*10 Assure correct dressing
- The dressing should be changed only by trained dialysis staff[2]. Conly et al. found less infection with gauze than with transparent dressing[24], but the question whether gauze should be preferred to transparent dressings remains unsolved[13].
- Especially in high-risk S. aureus nasal carriers (see below), topical povidone iodine ointment reduces exit site infections (0 % vs. 24 %), catheter tip colonisation (12 % vs. 42 %) and bacteraemia (0 % vs. 29 %) compared to the control group without povidone iodine ointment[25]. This ointment, however, might degrade catheters made of silicone[26].
- The use of povidone is contraindicated with silicone catheters due to the risk of damaging the silicone.

*11 Catheter Lock
- Locking the catheter, e.g. by heparin, to preserve patency between the dialysis sessions is routinely performed[27].
- An elevated risk of bleeding has been described, especially if the volume of the heparin lock was not adapted to the catheter size[28].
- Some authors recommend the use of a heparin lock as loading dose for the next dialysis session, reducing not only costs but also avoiding blood wastage[29]. In general, this procedure is performed without any complications, but it might risk embolisation of thrombus or of infected catheter content.
- Sodium citrate, polygeline, or urokinase are possible alternatives to heparin[28, 30]. In a comparison of heparin to 30 % trisodium citrate solution both were found to be equally effective in preventing thrombus formation in the catheter during the interdialysis period[31].
- There are potential risks to concentrated sodium citrate, e.g. bleeding, sodium overload, alkalosis due to the degradation of citrate by the liver, and changes in calcium concentration.
- In using an antimicrobial lock solution (Neutrolin®), blood stream infections were 0.2 / 1,000 catheter days, and no catheter was lost in 41 patient-years of treatment due to infection[32].
- To prevent both catheter thrombosis and infection, the combination of heparin with antibiotics was studied in vitro by Vercaigne et al.[33]. A mixture of heparin 5000 IU/ml with 10 mg/ml of cefazolin or 5 mg/ml of gentamycin retains bactericidal activity for 72 hours. Ciprofloxacin cannot be mixed with heparin, as it precipitates immediately. A mixture of 10 – 20 % trisodium citrate plus 2.3 mg/ml gentamicin used for locking the catheter was also successfully tested[34].
- Nevertheless the routine use of a prophylactic antibiotic lock solution cannot be recommended because of the potential risk of encouraging bacterial resistance. The prophylactic use of antimicrobial lock solutions such as Neutrolin needs further investigation.

*12 Treat nasal carrier of S. aureus
- About 52 – 57 % of all dialysis patients are nasal carrier of S. aureus[35, 36]. As they are at increased risk for catheter infection, all patients with catheters should be screened for S. aureus and eradication should be considered[2].
- The risk of infection can be reduced by the application of mupirocin at the exit site or by intranasal application[37]. Nasal mupirocin treatment in unselected dialysis pa-

tients led to eradication of nasal S. aureus in 96.3 % of the patients. The incidence of S. aureus bacteraemia was reduced fourfold.

***13 Monitor catheter**
- Catheter monitoring is mandatory to ensure dialysis efficacy and to prevent catheter-related hazards (see Algorithm: "Identification and management of permanent tunneled catheter dysfunction").
- In order to detect catheter-related infections early, the skin exit site should be examined at each haemodialysis treatment for signs of inflammation or tunnel track infections (erythema, pain, secretions, crusts, abscess). Regular measurement of body temperature, CRP and white blood cell counts are required to detect latent catheter contamination, which may be revealed by acute onset of bacteraemia during the dialysis session. Some experts also recommend periodic blood cultures through the catheter.
- Catheter dysfunction should be detected early and corrected to prevent dialysis inadequacy. Several observations may indicate a catheter dysfunction: a reduction in effective blood flow delivered (computed from the dialysis monitor), in the total amount of blood processed and dialysis dose delivered during the session, permanently or intermittently reduced blood flow rates and/or higher or lower than expected arterial or venous pressures. These signs may be caused by partial or complete catheter obstruction by host vein thrombosis or fibrin sleeves wrapping around the catheter tip. A catheterogram and/or venography are required to identify and visualise the precise cause.
- Inversion of the inlet and outlet lines of a twin central venous catheter leads to an increase in recirculation, thus reducing dialysis efficiency[38].

References see p. 136

Postoperative Control of A/V Fistula and Graft Function (1)

Patient with new A/V fistula or graft

Postoperative assessment vascular of access

Surgeon *1:
- Evaluation in recovery room and prior to discharge or after 2 d
- First outpatient evaluation within 10 days after surgery:
  - Stethoscopic examination of fistula or graft or use handheld Doppler
  - Check for signs of infection: pain, pus, swelling, erythema (hospitalisation, antibiotic treatment)
  - Exclusion of haematoma, thrombosis and bleeding
  - Check function of the hand
  - Check peripheral circulation: ischaemia, pain
  - Remove suture if necessary (if available, use absorbable suture)

Patient education *2:
- Check for pain, bleeding, haematoma formation
- Stethoscopic examination of fistula or graft by patient (if possible)
- Treatment of access site *3
- Recommendations concerning access arm *4

Nephrologist and staff *5:
Clinical assessment of vascular access 4 weeks after surgery:
- Evaluate fistula / graft function

Early infection present

- yes → **Management**

  Anastomotic infection *6:
  - Immediate hospitalisation
  - Blood culture, skin swab
  - Antibiotic treatment for 2 - 4 wk
  - Fistula: appropriate surgical intervention *7
  - Graft: remove immediately *8
  - Place catheter for dialysis

- no → Go to: Postoperative Control of A/V Fistula and Graft Function (2)

Postoperative Control of A/V Fistula and Graft Function (1)
*1 Surgeon
- Immediate postoperative evaluation comprises palpation of peripheral pulses and arterio-venous thrill. Auscultation may fail to detect arterio-venous murmur in tiny vessels – a frequent phenomenon in children. Doppler examination is then necessary to exclude early failure. The absence of murmur in adults in most cases indicates early failure. Haematoma or haemorrhage have to be excluded as well as peripheral ischaemia and neurological impairment, which may indicate steal syndrome. Development of acute ischaemic monomelic neuropathy, especially after creation of an elbow fistula in a diabetic patient, needs to be recognised.
- Wound healing should be complete after the first week. Therefore, a surgical examination within 10 days is useful to exclude skin necrosis, infection, and to remove sutures, if necessary, and assess fistula patency. At this time, a thrill should be palpable, and a murmur heard during auscultation. Again thorough assessment of the peripheral circulation and sensorimotor function of the hand is necessary, if the patient complains of symptoms of steal syndrome.

*2 Patient education
- The well informed, well prepared patient is the best partner. Patients should be trained to monitor the function of their vascular access daily. This self-assessment training can be performed by a nurse or a technician in one training session, supplemented by brochures and videos. The use of a diary may be helpful to ensure patient compliance.
- Patients should be taught to feel the pulse and thrill in their A/V fistula or graft. Simple palpation can reveal differences in intravascular pressure, indicating early development of aneurysm and stenosis. If possible, the patient should be instructed to use a stethoscope for auscultation of the vascular access. They should look for redness, swelling, new or changing pseudoaneurysms or evidence of pustule formation and report any development of pain. Abnormalities or changes should be brought to the attention of the patients' care team.

*3 Treatment of access site
- Patients should be taught how to wash the skin with soap and water daily and before dialysis.
- They should be advised to check that the cannulation site is rotated, except for the use of the buttonhole technique, see algorithm "Routine management of A/V fistula and graft" ***17**.

*4   Use of access arm
- Patients should be advised to avoid high pressure on their access site caused by occlusive clothes, by sleeping on the access arm or during compression of the bleeding access at the end of dialysis[1].
- They must avoid carrying heavy items with the access arm[1].

*5 Nephrologist and staff
- Clinical signs such as pain, redness, swelling, haematoma, intravascular pressure etc. can be obtained routinely by history, inspection, palpation and auscultation.
- Routine computer-assisted documentation of all access-relevant data should be available in the future and include reports of all surgical and interventional procedures, results of ultrasonographic and radiological diagnostic investigations and

the routinely documented data, such as arterial and venous pressure, during dialysis therapy. Trends should be monitored automatically.

*6 Management of anastomotic infection
- In forearm A/V fistulas and grafts, wound infection always means anastomotic infection with the risk of erosion and bleeding. Patients with signs and symptoms of infection following access creation should be immediately hospitalised and consequently treated.

*7 A/V Fistula: surgical intervention
- In A/V fistulas, uncomplicated infection without false aneurysm or bleeding (confirmed by colour-coded duplex-ultrasound) can be treated with antibiotics alone. In case of systemic signs of infection, excessive discharge of pus or progressive skin necrosis, early surgical wound revision is indicated.
- False aneurysms or active bleeding urge immediate surgical exploration of the anastomosis. The surgeon has to decide whether suturing the infective dehiscence of the anastomosis is possible or whether resection of the anastomosis with reconstruction of the artery is necessary[2].

*8 Graft: surgical intervention
- Following graft implantation, wound infection means infection of the complete graft and of both anastomoses. Antibiotic treatment alone is not likely to eliminate the infective agent. Hence a complete removal of the foreign body is advisable before local or systemic complications occur. The artery can be reconstructed by vein patching at the anastomotic site, the vein may be ligated proximally and distally to the anastomosis unless it is the main draining vein of the respective extremity[3]. A more conservative approach by leaving small cuffs of the graft on the artery and vein as patches, has also been performed successfully in those cases where the infection does not involve the anastomosis[3, 4, 5, 6].

References see p. 138

Postoperative control (2)

Postoperative Control of A/V Fistula and Graft Function (2)

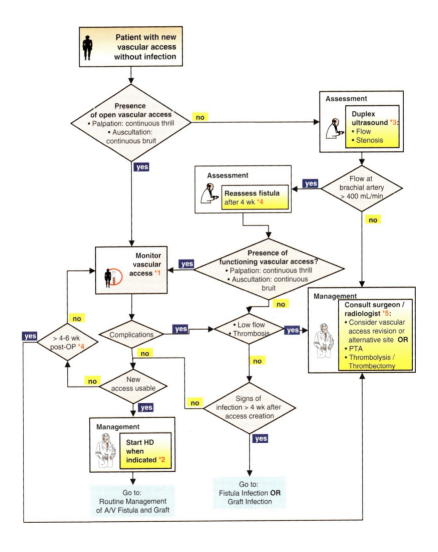

Postoperative Control of A/V Fistula and Graft Function (2)
*1 Monitor Vascular Access
- In native A/V fistulas, monitoring of the vascular access is important to assess maturation status (dilatation of the fistula sufficient to allow safe needling for dialysis by nurses or other appropriately trained healthcare workers) and to determine the ideal time for first cannulation. Native fistulas need time to mature. However, the decision when to cannulate first should be made individually on clinical assessment of vein diameter and topography.
- In general, A/V fistulas mature within 4-6 weeks. Tautenhahn et al. described a shorter average maturation time of three weeks[1]. Immature fistulas have fragile veins, are difficult to cannulate and provide insufficient blood flow[2]. Failure of maturation is higher in arteries with < 40 ml/min blood flow before fistula creation[3], but it is not influenced by the direction of blood flow (antegrade, retrograde) in the distal artery after creation of the fistula[4].
- A stenosis was found in all fistulas with delayed maturation in the study of Turmel-Rodrigues et al.[5]. Dilatation of the stenosis was successfully performed in 97 % of the cases, leading to a primary patency rate of nearly 40 % and a secondary patency rate of 75 % after one year. Further confirmation of these exceptional findings is required.
- Faiyaz et al. successfully salvaged 15 out of 17 A/V fistulas with delayed maturation by percutaneous ligation of accessory veins[6]. Whilst this procedure maybe of benefit in some cases, such high success with branch ligation is unusual. If a stenosis is the reason for non-maturation, it must be treated. In many cases of inadequate maturation, the problem is a critically reduced arterial inflow, particularly in patients with atherosclerotic disease. On the other hand, venous side branches can form a venous resource over time, a source for surgical repair as patch material, homologous interposition graft and other possibilities. To destroy a venous branch requires considerable reflection and should only be performed after consultation with an experienced surgeon.
- Konner published his single-centre experience of 748 consecutive primary direct arteriovenous accesses, of which only 52 % were located in the forearm. Without a single side branch ligated, he observed 99.4 % (96.8 %) functioning fistulae at four weeks in diabetic (non-diabetic) patients, and during a 1 – 7 year follow-up of his patients he found thrombosis rates as low as 0.03/patient year (0.07/patient year)[7].
- In grafts, postoperative swelling should have disappeared before the first cannulation. PTFE grafts should not be used routinely until 14 days after placement[8]. Normally, there will be no doubt about the quality of blood flow rates
- In both native A/V fistulas and grafts, the decision when to cannulate first time has to be made very carefully. Otherwise, the vascular access as well as the patient's confidence can be damaged substantially. In many cases, the problem does not arise from cannulation, but from subcutaneous bleeding and formation of haematoma after removal of the cannulas.

*2 Start HD when indicated
- The start of HD is indicated if GFR falls below 15 ml/min (UK < 10 ml/min) and there is one or more of the following signs: uncontrollable hypertension, fluid overload, malnutrition or uraemic symptoms. In any case, HD should be instituted before the GFR has fallen to 6 ml/min/1.73 m^2 [9]. High risk patients, e.g. diabetics, may benefit from an earlier start[9].

*3 Duplex ultrasound
- Due to maturation of an A/V fistula, the blood flow in the arm vessels augments 10 to 20 fold from baseline levels. In well-functioning radiocephalic A/V fistulas flows from 500 to 900 ml/min or higher may be found. In grafts and in upper arm A/V fistulas higher flows are obtained, ranging from 800-1400 ml/min. The maturation and increase in blood flow in native A/V fistulas is gradual and due to remodelling or adaptation of the vessel. After 4 - 6 weeks, radiocephalic A/V fistulas should have matured and be usable for haemodialysis.
- Failure to mature is usually due to insufficient blood flow, caused by a stenosis occurring anywhere from the subclavian artery to the outflow vein of the fistula. Blood flow of the radial artery measured by duplex ultrasound one and seven days after the operation may predict maturation. Low blood flow rates and velocities in the native fistula within the first 2 weeks usually result in fistula failure[10, 11]. A radial artery cross-sectional area of > 8.5 mm^2 and venous outflow of > 425 ml/min have a positive predictive value of 0.95 and 0.97, respectively, for the outcome of radiocephalic A/V fistulas[12].
- In a prospective study, Wong et al. measured blood flow velocity at 24 hours after fistula creation and found a significant difference between successful (average blood flow velocity of 0.53 m/s) and poor (average velocity 0.18 m/s) fistulas[11]. Also, duplex scan at 3 weeks revealed clear differences in blood flow and vein diameter between successful and poor fistulas. A combination of the two investigations should give a good clinical likelihood of successful maturation of the fistula and help expedite further investigation to improve fistula flow, surgical fistula revision or angioplasty, or create a more proximal fistula.

*4 Reassess fistula after 4 weeks
- A native A/V fistula generally matures within 4 - 6 weeks. Maturation of ulnar-basilic fistulas has been reported to take longer (6 weeks), but maturation time depends on the initial diameter of vein and artery and haemodynamic factors. In case of delayed maturation, an underlying stenosis must be looked for either by colour-coded duplex-ultrasound or by angiography.
- Cannulation and catheterisation of an immature fistula can generate stenosis[13].

*5 Consult surgeon / radiologist
- In cases of stenosis and, depending on their location, either surgery or angioplasty may be indicated. For planning and performing the appropriate treatment close co-operation between surgeon, nephrologist and radiologist as a team is needed[14].
- For arterial inflow stenoses and venous stenoses in the prospective needling segment and more centrally, angioplasty is indicated. In one study by Turmel-Rodrigues et al. an underlying stenosis was identified as the cause of dysmaturation in all cases. Treatment by interventional radiology led to a secondary patency rate of 79 % at one year[5]. However, haemodynamics of the A/V fistula as well as quality of inflow artery or outflow vein dictate maturation.
- Preference should be given to surgical intervention for isolated stenoses close to the anastomosis of a wrist fistula, where proximal re-anastomosis is likely to give better results than PTA. If the A/V fistula fails because of tiny or heavily calcified arteries, a decision may be made to create a more proximal A/V fistula connected to a larger artery.

References see p. 138

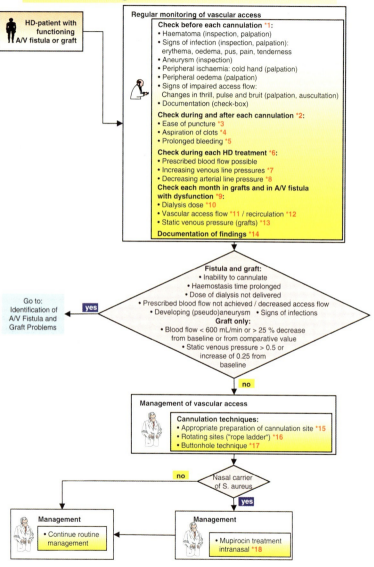

Routine Management of A/V Fistula and Graft

*1 Checks before each cannulation

- Inspection of the access site for signs of infection (redness, discharge, oedema), aneurysms, haematoma and colour (red, blue, white) of the hand is important for the early diagnosis of impending complications[1]. Swelling due to venous hypertension and the potential progression of acral necrosis should be monitored prior to haemodialysis treatment. Venous dilatations and aneurysms in grafts without stenosis (low pressure aneurysms) can be cannulated using the lateral side provided that the skin is completely healthy.
- Palpation along the access site from its arterial anastomosis up to the outflow veins may give an idea of the function of the access. In fistulas normally a strong thrill and weak pulsation is felt. In grafts the presence of a good thrill is associated with flows of > 450 ml/min[2]. The intravascular pressure should be equal at any segment. Differences in intravascular pressure and an increase in pulsation indicates an outflow stenosis. In fistulas a stenosis can be felt along the access tract by palpation. Palpation of peripheral pulses (radial and ulnar at the wrist) is indicated in patients with hand perfusion disturbances (white/blue hand). However, in one third of proximal procedures with the brachial artery as in flow artery there is no distal pulse as a consequence of a mild non limb-threatening steal 3. Digital pressure or wrist-to-brachial pressure index measurements could be used instead. An index > 0.5 or a digital pressure > 50 mm Hg rules out a limb threatening steal [3, 4].
- Auscultation normally reveals a typical thrill with a long diastolic component that is shortened in case of haemodynamically relevant stenosis. A stenosis causes a high-pitch bruit. In thrombosis, there will be no bruit at all.
- In patients with grafts, palpation may be difficult due to the deep subcutaneous position of the graft. Auscultation is more reliable and should concentrate on the venous outflow tract for detection of graft-to-vein anastomotic stenosis.

*2 Check during and after each cannulation

- Difficulties in access cannulation or prolonged bleeding should be documented in the patients' medical records and addressed by the medical team[5].

*3 Ease of puncture

- After overcoming the initial resistance of the access wall, the fistula needle should be easily advanced into the access. Further resistance may indicate that the needle is not within the access lumen or that it may have entered the back wall. Resistance can also indicate the presence of pseudo-intimal hyperplasia or thrombus.

*4 Aspiration of clots

- Aspiration of clots suggests impending thrombosis and is an indication for further access evaluation (measurement of access flow, imaging by ultrasound or angiography). However, aspiration of clots might also be caused by improper placement of the needle. Thus, puncture should be repeated. Clot aspiration is not an indication for anti-platelet or anti-thrombotic agents.

*5 Prolonged bleeding

- Prolonged bleeding should raise suspicion of high intra-access pressure, outflow (downstream) stenosis or local inflammation. Clinical examination of the site should be performed and previous static or dynamic venous pressure measurements should be reviewed. Measurements of access flow and of static or dynamic venous pressures should be performed during the next treatment as true outflow stenosis means impending thrombosis. However, prolonged bleeding may also be caused by excessive heparinisation of the blood circuit, access laceration during previous cannulation or skin atrophy.

*6 **Checks during each HD treatment**
- Evidence of access dysfunction can be observed during haemodialysis. Access recirculation, the return of processed blood from the venous needle back up through the arterial needle, can sometimes be observed during dialysis. Recirculation usually occurs when the access flow is lower than the prescribed pump flow (Q_b)[6]. Recirculation is more commonly seen in A/V fistulas than in PTFE grafts, because grafts tend to clot more rapidly when access flow is less than 600 – 800 ml/min[7, 8, 9]. A/V fistulas, however, usually remain patent even with access flow of less than 400 ml/min.
- Information about possible access dysfunction can be obtained during dialysis by occluding the A/V fistula or graft between the two dialysis needles. In the presence of outflow stenosis, particularly in grafts, venous pressure will rise and arterial pressure may fall. With arterial inflow disease, arterial pressure will fall while venous will remain the same during inter-needle compression[10].

*7 **Increasing venous line pressures**
- Elevated dynamic or static venous pressures (see **13**) are indicative of possible venous outflow stenosis in grafts. However, McDougal et al. found no significant difference in the venous pressure in failed grafts or in grafts that did not fail at blood flow rates of 200 ml/min and 400 ml/min. They concluded, that single static or dynamic venous pressure monitoring was not predictive of graft failure[11]
- Dynamic venous pressure is measured during the first five minutes of the dialysis session (for procedure: see appendix). Dynamic venous pressure repeatedly >150 mm Hg with 16-gauge needle at 200 – 225 ml/min-blood flow may be indicative of possible venous outflow stenosis[12]. Thus monthly access monitoring should be anticipated.
- Dynamic pressures are less useful in A/V fistulas than in grafts. Due to their multiplicity of run-off veins, the venous pressure may not rise with outflow stenosis. Upper arm A/V fistulas behave more like PTFE grafts because of their singular venous outflow.

*8 **Decreasing arterial line pressures**
- Decreasing pre-pump arterial pressure (= high negative pressure) over time (weeks) is another indication of decreased access flow and access dysfunction. Although this can be inferred by noting a collapsed arterial pillow, the measurement of pre-pump arterial pressure is preferable. When the pre-pump arterial pressure is < 150 to – 250 mm Hg, the blood pump is no longer able to deliver the prescribed Q_b[13]. This is frequently an indication of inflow disease in A/V fistulas and PTFE grafts. These high negative pre-pump pressures also correlate with development of haemolysis[14]. If the negative arterial pressure is below –150 mm Hg, the dangerously high negative aspirating pressure inside the vascular access might also damage the access wall.

*9 **Checks each month in grafts and in A/V fistulas with dysfunction**
- Regardless of the mode of monitoring, most investigators have found significant

and cost effective improvements of up to 70 % in cumulative access patency, when prospective monitoring techniques are combined with early correction of stenosis using either angioplasty or surgical revision[12, 15, 16, 17, 18, 19]. Thus these monitoring regimens also help to reduce costs as maintenance of vascular access accounts for 17 – 25 % of all hospitalisations in dialysis patients in the USA[16].

- Screening procedures include physical examination[2], measurement of vascular access flow (Qa), of recirculation, of static and dynamic venous pressure (VP) and colour-coded duplex ultrasound. Monitoring of venous pressure, blood flow or both and intervention in cases of stenoses reduces thrombosis rates to < 0.5 events per patient year, i.e. below the quality recommendation of the DOQI guideline[16, 20].
- It is recommended that each unit uses one or more monthly screening tests to monitor vascular access performance in order to predict complications. Unfortunately, the prediction of impending vascular access thrombosis, using one or a combination of simple tests, performed whenever possible during the regular dialysis treatment, is still not perfect. The predictive power is poorer when using a single measurement instead of a trend analysis, or a single technique instead of a combination of parameters[11]. Vascular access flow is probably the most useful and reliable parameter available, especially if performed serially[21].

*10 Dialysis dose
- Low delivered dialysis dose might be indicative of either insufficient blood flow or high recirculation, possibly due to stenosis. However, recirculation by itself is a relative insensitive parameter, detecting stenosis very late[22].

*11 Vascular access flow Q_a
Direct measurement of access blood flow (Q_a)
- Q_a determination is considered the best method to monitor vascular access function and predict vascular access failure[17, 21, 23, 24]. Moreover, trend analysis of serial Q_a determinations are more effective than a single measurement.
- Q_a can be determined by Doppler ultrasound[15] or dilution methods (e.g. haematocrit dilution, thermodilution, conductivity (ionic) dilution)[25, 26, 27, 28] (see appendix).
- It is still controversial whether Q_a should be measured only at the beginning of the dialysis session, with stable blood pressure conditions, as vascular access flow may vary over the course of the treatment especially in patients with haemodynamic instability. While Rehman et al. recommend measurement of Q_a only during the first 90 minutes of the dialysis session[29], Agharazii et al. found only a non-significant drop in Q_a during the haemodialysis session of fifty patients[30].
- Angiography should be performed when access flow falls below certain cut-off values. However, it still remains unknown which cut-off value should be used. Cut-off values differ from 500 to 600 ml/min in native A/V fistulas and 650 to 800 ml/min in grafts, or a reduction of Q_a of 20-25 %[17, 18, 31]. These differences were to some extent due to using different measurement techniques.
- Neyra et al. found a high risk of thrombosis if Q_a decreased by 15 %. Reduction in access blood flow of 35 % increased the risk of thrombosis almost 14-fold compared to accesses with no decrease in blood flow[23].
- However, other authors could not confirm the benefits of a vascular access surveillance program. Paulson et al. found no association between future thrombosis and Q_a, or decrease in Q_a[32, 33]. Neither static nor dynamic venous pressure

predicted stenosis. Q_a was only a poor predictor of stenosis[11]. While Wang could find an association between low Q_a (< 500 mL/min) and an elevated risk of thrombosis in grafts, this association was not found with A/V fistulas[34].

- Lumsden et al. used duplex ultrasound to detect stenosis > 50 % in ePTFE grafts. Considering the high costs of prophylactic surveillance with duplex ultrasound and the absence of improved patency rates found in their study, Lumsden et al. questioned the use of this technique in grafts[35].

*12 Measurement of recirculation

- Recirculation is less popular as a screening technique since it detects stenosis relatively late at a critical stage. Moreover, its predictive value is especially poor in grafts[36]. It is more useful in A/V fistulas provided that the two needles are placed in a segment of the fistula vein without side branches and collaterals (see ***13**) (for performance of measurement and formula, see appendix).

*13 Static intra-access venous pressure (SVP)

- Static venous pressure is less accurate in A/V fistulas than in grafts, as in the former, collateral vessels might be present or develop, preventing a marked increase in venous pressure[36] (for procedure and formula see appendix). Static venous pressure should be measured every two weeks in grafts.
- However, even in grafts, static venous pressure is not an optimal screening method to predict future thrombosis. For a threshold of $SPR_v \geq 0.4$ in grafts, sensitivity and specificity of the predictive value for thrombosis within one month was 73 % and 47 %, respectively. With a threshold of $SPR_v \geq 0.5$, it was 48 % and 75 %, respectively[37].
- A guide for interpreting the pressures measured, according to the DOQI-guidelines, is given in table 3.

Table 3:
Interpretation of the normalized, arterial and venous static intra-access pressures

	Graft		A/V fistula	
	SPR_a	SPR_v	SPR_a	SPR_v
Normal	0.35-0.74	0.15-0.49	0.13-0.43	0.08-0.34
Venous outlet Stenosis	> 0.75 or	> 0.5 or	> 0.43 or	> 0.35
Intra-access Stenosis	> 0.75 and	< 0.5 or	> 0.43 and	< 0.35
Arterial inflow Stenosis	< 0.3	–	< 0.13	–

SPR_a = ratio of normalised arterial static intra-access pressure to mean arterial pressure (see appendix)
SPR_v = ratio of normalised venous static intra-access pressure to mean arterial pressure (see appendix)

*14 Summary of access monitoring

- Prospective surveillance of grafts to look for stenosis, malfunction and pre-emptive correction probably improves patency rates and life expectancy of the access. In the absence of a gold standard method with high sensitivity and specificity for surveillance and prevention of vascular access failure, each unit should establish its own quality assurance program to monitor prospectively their vascular

Routine Management of A/V Fistula and Graft

accesses, combining more than one isolated test (see appendix 2 for proposal of check box).
- There is no evidence that surveillance of autogenous AV fistulas is cost effective.

*15 Appropriate preparation of cannulation site
- In order to reduce the risk of infection and bacteraemia, the cannulation site should be cautiously prepared, according to standards (e.g. as given in the European Best Practice Guidelines – Haemodialysis)[38].
- The needle site should be palpated before preparation of the skin. After cleaning the skin with warm water and soap, chlorhexidine should be applied to the skin in the region of cannulation, as it is considered to be a better antiseptic than povidone iodine. If povidone iodine is used, it should be applied for at least 2 – 3 minutes to allow it to dry. Alcohol (70 %) can be used in patient who have side-effects with the other antiseptics. It should be applied for at least one minute. Wearing new gloves for every patient is mandatory.
- In using the buttonhole technique (see ***16** below), puncturing through the scab should be avoided, as this may introduce germs into the access and also cause the needle to puncture and destroy the sides of the tunnel. The scab has to be removed by a different, sterile cannula, before the access can be punctured.

*16 Rotating sites ("rope ladder")
- The basic knowledge of the types of repeated cannulation were developed by Krönung[39]. In most patients with A/V fistulas the "rope ladder" technique is the favoured technique. In A/V fistulas, the rotating cannulation sites cause a regular, but moderate dilatation of the vein.
- Cannulation of only a small area of the access ("area cannulation") by gradually weakening the access wall causes aneurysms in A/V fistulas and pseudo-aneurysms in grafts, thus destroying the latter. Therefore, this technique should be abandoned.

*17 Buttonhole technique
- The "buttonhole" technique, which has been used exclusively in A/V fistulas, is still discussed controversially. In this technique, also called "constant-site" method, the vascular access is always punctured at the same place, with the same angle, using the same "tunnel" for the cannula. Over time, the tissue around the needle becomes scared, thus directing the needle to the vascular access. It seems to be a good alternative for experienced hands[40, 41].
- The buttonhole technique is recommended for self-cannulation. Dull needles have been developed, which reduce the risk of damaging the scared tunnel while cannulating the access. These dull needles can be used after the tunnel has been created. With the buttonhole technique, less bleeding, less pain and less cannulation failure have been reported (see appendix for details of performance).

*18 Mupirocin treatment intranasal
- Patients with nasal carriage of S. aureus are at an increased risk of bacteraemia caused by S. aureus. The infection rate can be reduced fourfold by the eradication of S. aureus by nasal mupirocin treatment[42].
- The European Best Practice Guidelines recommend screening all patients with a past history of S. aureus infection and to consider intervention[38].

References see p. 139

Identification of A/V Fistula and Graft Problems

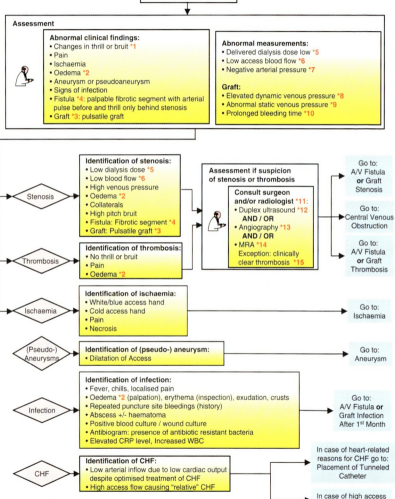

Identification of A/V Fistula and Graft Problems

*1 Changes in thrill or bruit
- Vascular access flow is regarded as an important indicator of future patency and can be screened by clinical examination. The patients themselves should either listen for bruit or palpate for thrill and/or pulse daily. Patients with a palpable thrill at the arterial, mid and venous segment of a graft usually have an access blood flow of > 450 ml/min[1].
- The bruit should be assessed with regard to its continuous character and diastolic component. Shortening of the diastolic part is found in the presence of stenosis. Intensification of the bruit may indicate stenosis or stricture. A significant decrease in bruit after elevation of the arm may be a symptom of reduced arterial inflow, in some patients caused by hypotension without an underlying morphological alteration.
- In cases of graft outflow obstruction, Doppler investigation produces a "waterhammer" like sound. This is not audible in thrombosed grafts.

*2 Oedema
- Oedema may be an indicator of infection or venous outflow impairment. The pattern of the oedema and the type of collateralisation can reveal a relatively exact location of the venous obstruction.
- Isolated forearm oedema may occur in distal arteriovenous access with stenosis of the main draining forearm vein.
- A swelling of the total upper extremity (sometimes combined with reddening similar to cellulitis and ulceration) signals a central venous stenosis. Its location may be in the subclavian vein, caused by previous catheterisation, or particularly in the left brachiocephalic (innominate) vein with a retrograde filling of the internal jugular vein, often with drainage via the contralateral internal jugular vein.
- Obstruction of the innominate vein or superior vena cava may cause breast and face-swelling, sometimes even headaches due to benign intracranial hypertension.
- Any case of oedema requires careful clinical examination, in most cases supplemented by ultrasonography and other radiological investigations.

*3 Pulsatility
- In access graft stenosis, clinical examination is of limited value. Grafts with a thrill all over are unlikely to have a flow of less than 450 ml/min1. Palpable graft pulsation, however, is predictive of venous anastomotic stenosis and consequently reduced flow only in 28 % of cases[1].
- Pulsatility is also be encountered in stenosis of A/V fistulas.

*4 Fistula
- Due to the superficial course of the access vein, thorough clinical examination alone is sufficient to plan the intervention in most cases of A/V fistula stenosis[2]. In anastomotic venous stenosis, the fibrotic segment of the vein can easily be palpated. Imaging by colour-coded duplex ultrasonography, angiography or MRA is indicated if an additional arterial stenosis is suspected, when arterial pulse at the anastomosis is reduced or lost. Stenosis within the punctured segment of the vein causes a strong pulse in the most peripheral segment of the vein without a murmur, a high-frequency thrill and a weak murmur proximal to the stenosis. Junctional stenosis, located in the superficial vein above the punctured segment and close to its

junction with the draining deep vein, causes pulsation of the whole superficial vein and sometimes development of excessive superficial collaterals. On arm elevation, the prestenotic vein will not collapse. [Pre-treatment colour-coded duplex-ultrasonography or fistulography is necessary in junctional stenoses (see **11**)].

*5 **Delivered dialysis dose low**
- Decreases in delivered dialysis dose, as measured by Kt/V or URR, may be indicative of either insufficient blood flow or high recirculation, possibly due to stenosis. However, recirculation is a relatively insensitive parameter, detecting stenosis very late[3].

*6 **Low access blood flow**
- Progressive stenosis due to intimal hyperplasia, usually at the site of the A/V anastomosis in native A/V fistulas and venous anastomosis in grafts, jeopardises the blood flow with subsequent thrombotic occlusion. Therefore, it seems clear, that there is need to follow A/V fistulas and grafts in a standardised surveillance program with special emphasis on vascular access flow (Q_a) measurements. Several studies stress the importance of non-invasive or in-line flow measurements and correlate these with the outcome of native A/V fistulas and grafts.
- Thrombosis rates in grafts were 92.8 % and 26.3 % when the access flow was < 800 or > 1600 ml/min, respectively[4]. The mean flow in grafts, that did not thrombose, compared to grafts, that thrombosed, was 1193 vs 875 ml/min as measured by ultrasound dilution technique (1171 ml/min vs 762 ml/min measured by Doppler ultrasound). The relative risk was 1.23, 1.67, and 2.39 with a Q_a of 950, 650 and 300 ml/min[5]. Half of the accesses clotted, when Qa was less than 750 ml/min, while only 2 out of 27 accesses clotted with Q_a > 750 ml/min[6]. Depner documented high failure rate from stenosis and thrombosis in accesses with Q_a < 600 ml/min, while those with flows > 800 ml/min had few failures[7].
- With a cut-off value of 600 ml/min the rate of thrombosis was 7.2 for the patients having a Q_a < 600 ml/min compared to those patients having a Q_a > 600 ml/min[8]. Grafts with Qa < 500 ml/min had a relative risk of clotting within 8 weeks of 3.12, compared to grafts with Q_a of 1100 – 1400 ml/min[9].
- Tonelli et al. investigated 177 native A/V fistulas[10]. They used ultrasound dilution technique to determine blood flow Q_a. In fistulas with a blood flow rate < 500 ml/min, a subclinical stenosis was found in 81 % of cases (defined as a > 50 % reduction of vessel diameter determined by angiography). Thus, the authors suggested use of a blood flow rate of 500 ml/min as a cut off value, corresponding to the recommendation of the Canadian Society of Nephrology[11].
- As these different results indicate, it is difficult to determine a fixed cut-off value, because the blood flow rates of accesses that thrombose overlap with the blood flow rates of the accesses that did not thrombose. In addition, native A/V fistulas have in general lower blood flow rates than grafts, despite a lower risk of thrombosis[12]. Wang et al. found that grafts had a 5.6 greater risk on thrombosis compared to native A/V fistulas[9].
- A single measurement of reduced intra-access blood flow appears to be a relatively poor predictor for thrombosis[13] the percentage of decrease in flow did, not correlate with the likelihood of access failure.
- Serial measurements with a documented decrease of blood flow over time seems more accurate than single measurements. In a prospective study, Neyra[14] observed a 13.6-fold increase in the relative risk of thrombosis for accesses with

more than 35 % decrease in vascular access blood flow when compared to those accesses with no changes in blood flow.
- Nevertheless, the DOQI guideline consider an absolute Q_a of < 600 ml/min or a decline in Q_a of > 25 % in vascular accesses with a Q_a > 1,000 ml/min between two monthly measurements as indicative of an enhanced risk of thrombosis[15].
- Gallego et al. concluded, that early detection of stenosis, indicated by increased venous pressure or by difficulties in cannulation, and subsequent treatment of the stenosis can prevent thrombosis[16].
- Schwab et al. initiated an active intervention program in grafts and A/V fistulas with flows < 600 ml/min or a decrease in flow of > 20 % compared to the last measurement. The overall thrombosis rate for grafts and A/V fistulas declined from 25 to 16 %. For A/V fistulas alone, the thrombosis rate decreased from 16 to 7 %[17].
- In a meta-analysis of 12 studies, Paulson et al. found a wide range of Qa values that were used as indicators for impending failure[13]. In combining these studies, the predictive value of flow measurement for thrombosis was 0.70 and for access failure 0.76. Serial Qa measurements are a better indicator than a single measurement.

*7 Negative arterial pressure
- With a standard 15-gauge needle set, the development of excessive negative pressures below –200 mm Hg in the arterial blood line at a blood flow rate of 400 ml/min indicates a failure of the fistula to provide the flow demanded by the blood pump. This means, that the fistula-flow from the anastomosis is inadequate[18, 19].

*8 Elevated dynamic venous pressure
- Dynamic venous pressure is considered abnormal when it is greater than 125 mmHg with a blood flow of 200 ml/min with the use of a 15 gauge needle on three repeated treatments[20] (for details: see appendix). Bosman et al. measured the venous drip chamber pressure, while the vascular access of the patient was placed at the same level as the venous drip chamber (thus avoiding false measurements due to differences in height between the drip chamber and the vascular access). Venous drip chamber pressure did not discriminate between patients with graft flow > or < 600 ml/min[8].
- Access flow (see ***6**) and static venous pressure (see ***9**) are more sensitive indicators of access dysfunction then dynamic venous pressure[8, 21, 22].

*9 Abnormal static venous pressure / static venous pressure ratio (SPRv)
- Static venous pressure (SVP) is measured with the blood flow stopped (for procedure see appendix II). It should be normalised to mean arterial blood pressure (MAP), thus yielding the quotient SVP/MAP, the "Static venous pressure ratio" (SPRv). However, intra-access venous pressure is not identical with venous drip chamber pressure but must be corrected for the differences in height between the drip chamber and the access. A vertical difference of 1 cm corresponds to a pressure change of approximately 0.75 mm Hg[23] (see appendix for calculation of SVP).
- Static venous pressure ratios in grafts are abnormal, if $SPR_v \geq 0.5$ or if an increase of 0.25 from baseline is seen within one month, for A/V fistulas, the threshold is $SPR_v \geq 0.35$[21, 24]. Besarab et al. found a sensitivity of 91 % and 48 % and a specificity of 86 % and 100 % in grafts and A/V fistulas, respectively, for 50 % luminal diameter reduction with a $SVP/MAP \geq 0.4$[21]. Static venous pressure is more effective than dynamic venous pressure for monitoring grafts[25].

Identification of A/V Fistula and Graft Problems

- For A/V fistulas, venous pressure is less effective in detecting stenosis, as collaterals permit blood-outflow without dramatic increase in venous pressure. In addition, stenosis in native A/V fistulas most commonly occur in the inflow or in the body of the fistula, thus the venous needle is usually placed after (or downstream of) the stenosis. In contrast, stenosis in grafts are frequently located in the outflow or at the venous anastomosis, thus the needle is placed before the stenosis. In the latter, the intra-access pressure increases and can be detected[26].

*10 Prolonged bleeding time
- Measurement and documentation of bleeding time after needle withdrawal (without excessive anticoagulation) has been mentioned as a further method (but not method of choice) to detect graft or fistula stenosis[12].
- Prolonged bleeding post dialysis for more than 10 minutes or a change from the patient's baseline in the absence of a change in anticoagulation may indicate outflow stenosis particularly in PTFE grafts, but can also occur in skin atrophy. Repeated prolonged bleeding is an indication for evaluation of the vascular access, to rule out venous outflow stenosis.
- Bleeding after removal of the needle is also dependent on the needle size and the degree of anticoagulation[27].

*11 Indications for imaging
- In cases of A/V fistula thrombosis, clinical examination may reveal the presence and location of an underlying stenosis in most patients.
- When a stenosis of an A/V fistula or graft is suspected, adequate and timely assessment should be performed to initiate early treatment before thrombosis[28]. The decision whether clinical examination alone is sufficient or additional ultrasound examination must be performed before stenosis treatment, depends on local custom and practice. In cases of endovascular treatment, pre-, intra-, and post-operative angiography take place as a matter of course. When open surgical revision is undertaken, completion angiography should also be performed whenever possible. Purely diagnostic angiography without concomitant treatment should be avoided in order to reduce inconvenience for the patient and treatment delay.
- Once thrombosis has occurred, immediate surgical or interventional radiological clot removal is necessary to allow for haemodialysis through the arterio-venous access without the need for central venous catheter insertion. Correction of the underlying stenosis is an integral part of any declotting procedure.

*12 Colour-coded duplex-sonography
- Whenever stenosis is suspected, colour-coded duplex ultrasonography can be performed to locate and to quantify the stenosis[29, 30]. Colour-coded duplex ultrasonography is able to replace angiography except for hand arteries and central veins[31].
- In cases of low flow or clinically obvious tight stenosis, duplex examination should be performed only if it does not delay PTA or surgical revision.
- Angiography is not necessary if colour-coded duplex-ultrasonography shows evidence of an isolated stenosis close to the anastomosis in forearm fistulas amenable to surgical revision by proximal re-anastomosis.
- Colour-coded duplex-ultrasonography can be helpful in defining the extent of thrombosis.

- Colour-coded duplex examination is especially valuable in detecting stenoses and flow measurements in immature fistulas of predialysis patients in whom iodine injection ought to be avoided.
- An Italian team has reported that it perform graft dilatations only under colour Doppler guidance[32].

*13 Angiography
- Isolated diagnostic angiography without concomitant dilatation or surgical revision must be avoided. Angiography is performed before, during and after dilatation or percutaneous declotting and after surgical thrombectomy in order to guide the treatment and document the final results.

*14 Magnetic resonance angiography (MRA)
- When central (mediastinal) vein stenosis or occlusion is suspected, angiography of the complete venous drainage up to the cavo-atrial junction is mandatory, because only the lateral half of the subclavian vein can be visualised by ultrasound[30]. Magnetic resonance angiography of the central chest veins is accurate and even superior to contrast venography, which fails to show all patent thoracic vessels[33, 34]. However, it is not yet, and may never be, possible to perform recanalisation procedures under MRA guidance.

*15 Exception: Clinically clear thrombosis
- Native A/V fistula and graft thrombosis must be treated without preceding diagnostic work-up. The underlying stenosis must be demonstrated (and treated) in combination with surgical or interventional clot removal.
- See: Management of A/V fistula / graft thrombosis for details.

References see p. 142

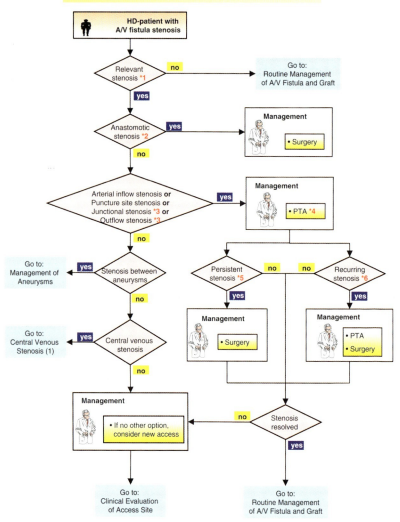

Management of A/V Fistula Stenosis

*1 Relevant stenosis
- Stenosis should be treated, if the reduction of diameter exceeds 50 % and is associated with abnormal physical findings, reduction in access flow, measured dialysis dose or previous thrombosis.
- A stenotic lesion or vessel segment, induced by intimal hyperplasia, is the most common cause for low flow. In radiocephalic A/V fistulas, 55 – 75 % of these stenoses are located at the A/V anastomosis and 25 % in the outflow tract[1, 2, 3]. In brachiocephalic and / or basilic A/V fistulas the typical location (55 %) is at the junction of the cephalic with the subclavian vein and the basilic with the axillary vein, respectively[1]. An arterial inflow stenosis > 2 cm from the anastomosis is rare but may jeopardise flow in the A/V fistula.

*2 Stenosis of the anastomotic area
- Primary surgical treatment is indicated in stenoses of the anastomotic area located in the lower forearm. However, PTA is also possible although its results are likely less durable.
- Primary interventional treatment is indicated in stenoses of the anastomotic area located in the upper forearm and in the upper arm. However, surgery must be considered in cases of early or repeated recurrences of the lesions.
- Dilatation or surgical revision of anastomotic stenoses in upper arm fistulas can result in steal syndrome and hand ischaemia. Prudent dilatation to 5 or 6 mm is recommended first and it is rarely indicated to dilate to more than 6 mm. Nephrologists must be warned to look after the hand of such patients in the days and weeks following the dilatations or surgical revisions.

*3 Outflow stenosis
- Percutaneous transluminal angioplasty (PTA) is the first treatment option in outflow vein (cephalic/basilic) stenosis (see appendix for details).
- Junctional stenosis, i.e. stenosis at the junction of the superficial vein with the deep venous system, can also be treated by PTA.
- Surgical correction may be needed after failed PTA with and without stent placement.
- An eventual stent placed in the final arch of the cephalic vein must not protrude into the subclavian vein where it could induce stenosis and preclude future use of the downstream (basilic, brachial, and axillary) veins.

*4 PTA
- In order to visualise the stenoses, angiography is performed by puncturing of the brachial artery in case of anastomotic problems or by direct puncture of the vein above the anastomosis if an outflow problem has occurred[4].
- It is controversial, whether long stenosis should be treated radiologically or surgically. While some authors recommend surgical intervention in long segment stenoses (longer than 6 cm)[5], either by graft interposition[6] or vein transposition, others recommend radiological intervention also in long stenoses (> 5 cm)[4]. Studies proving the superiority of one of the treatment are not available. However, some radiological series recently confirmed that long stenoses (> 2 cm) usually had a poorer outcome[7].

*5 **Persistent stenosis**
- Some stenoses cannot be dilated by balloon angioplasty. These "hard" stenoses can be treated with atherectomy devices or cutting balloons, first described by Vorwerk et al.[8].

*6 **Recurring stenosis**
- Recurring stenoses can be treated radiologically, with or without a stent, or surgically[4]. The decision should be made considering the individual situation of the patient and the invasiveness of surgical treatment.
- Despite complete opening of the PTA balloon (without waste) of sufficient diameter, the dilated vessel wall may collapse immediately after removal of the balloon. This elastic recoil can be treated with stent implantation, especially in central veins, as long as the ostia of major side branches will not be covered by the stent. There is no room for stent placement in the needling areas of forearm fistulas except for acute PTA-induced ruptures not controlled by a prolonged balloon inflation.

References see p. 144

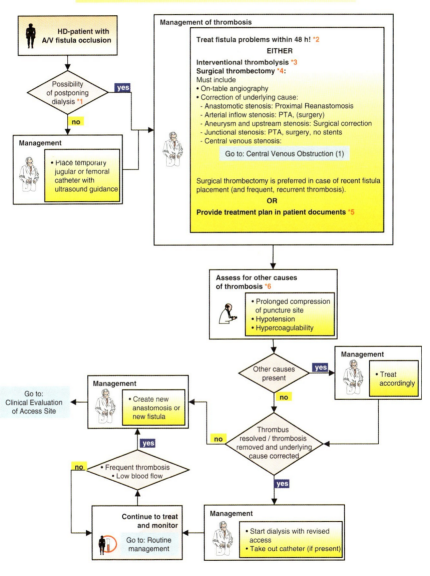

Management of A/V Fistula Thrombosis

*1 Postpone dialysis if possible
  - Postponement of dialysis might be possible in patients who are not expected to develop pulmonary oedema. Increase in body weight since the last dialysis session must be checked to assess amount of excess water. Furthermore, the patients must not show symptoms of uraemia, and the potassium level must not exceed 5.6 mmol/L.

*2 Treat fistula thrombosis within 48 hours whenever possible
  - The duration and site of A/V fistula thrombosis as well as the type of access are important determinants of treatment outcome. Fistula thrombosis should be treated without unnecessary delay. Early declotting allows an immediate use without need for central venous access. Thrombi become progressively fixed to the vein wall, which makes surgical extraction more difficult. Thrombosis may affect the postanastomotic vein segment as result of anastomotic stenosis or may begin at the needle site. When the clot is localised at the anastomosis in radiocephalic and brachiocephalic fistulas, the outflow vein may remain patent due to the natural sidebranches that continue to carry venous blood flow. In this type of clotting it is possible to create a new proximal anastomosis[1, 2] even after some days.
  - Thrombosis in A/V fistulas with transposed basilic veins usually leads to clot propagation of the entire vein.
  - Although comparative studies are missing, the available literature[3-13] strongly suggests that thrombosed autogenous A/V fistulas should preferably be treated by interventional radiology. The only exception may be forearm A/V fistulas thrombosed due to anastomotic stenosis. It is likely that in such cases, creation of a proximal new anastomosis will provide excellent results although no surgical series has ever demonstrated that to date. There remains a paucity of literature on the results of surgical intervention for fistula thrombosis although there are many papers confirming the success of radiological intervention.

*3 Interventional thrombolysis
  - Thrombolysis can be performed mechanically or pharmacomechanically. While the immediate success rate is higher in grafts than in A/V fistulas (99 % versus 93 % in forearm A/V fistulas), the primary patency rate of the forearm A/V fistula at one year is much higher (49 % versus 14 %). One year secondary patency rates are 80 % in forearm and 50 % in upper arm A/V fistulas, respectively[3].
  - In A/V fistulas, the combination of a thrombolytic agent (urokinase or plasminogen activator tPA) with balloon angioplasty resulted in immediate success rates of 94 %.
  - Liang et al. reported a success rate of 93 % and a primary patency rate at one year of 70 % in restoring flow of thrombosed forearm A/V fistulas by PTA[12].
  - Haage et al. performed 81 percutaneous treatments of thrombosed A/V fistulas[5]. Full flow restoration was achieved in 88.9 % of A/V fistulas, although primary one-year patency rate was only 26 %, overall one-year patency rate was 51 %.

*4 Surgical thrombectomy
  - Surgical thrombectomy is performed with an embolectomy catheter. In tortuous or aneurysmal veins, manual retrograde thrombus expression can be helpful.
  - On-table completion angiography of the reopened vein as well as the central venous outflow tract should be performed whenever possible to find/exclude addi-

tional stenoses or a persistent thrombus. Identification and simultaneous correction of the underlying cause(s) of thrombosis are integral parts of any surgical or interventional declotting procedure (see Algorithm "Management of A/V Fistula Stenosis", **1**).
- The best results of surgery probably will be encountered after proximal re-anastomosis for anastomotic stenosis of forearm A/V fistulas – which is indeed the most frequent location of stenosis in this type of access. Primary (secondary) patency of the new proximal anastomosis has been reported to be as high as 80 % (89 % – 95 %) at one year and 67 % (87 % – 89 %) at two years[2].

*5 **Provide treatment plan in patients document**
- Regular multidisciplinary meetings with nephrologists, dialysis nurses, surgeons and interventional radiologists are needed to establish a treatment plan for difficult or complicated vascular accesses. Adequate documentation of the outcome of these meetings, results of investigations, description of radiological and surgical interventions are of utmost importance. Ideally, a database should be used for this purpose. Information from the surgeon to the dialysis nurse, concerning the time and location of first cannulation of new / revised accesses, is to be incorporated in the treatment plan. If access failure recurs frequently in a short time period, a new fistula may need to be created[15].

*6 **Assess for other causes of thrombosis**
- The vast majority of access thrombosis is due to stenosis of the A/V fistula. Other causes such as post-dialysis hypotension, excessive dehydration, hypercoagulability (deficiency of AT3, protein S, antiphospholipid antibodies), trauma, or prolonged compression of the puncture site are probably only associated risk factors or triggers to reveal an underlying stenosis. Infection can also cause or be associated with access thrombosis.
- If prolonged compression of the puncture site is necessary, the patient should be taught how to compress it without occluding the vascular access. Mechanical devices should be avoided and haemostasis should be performed with a sterile gloved finger over a small haemostatic gauze. The nurse, the assistant nurse or the patient must feel the thrill under the finger during the tamponade.

References see p. 145

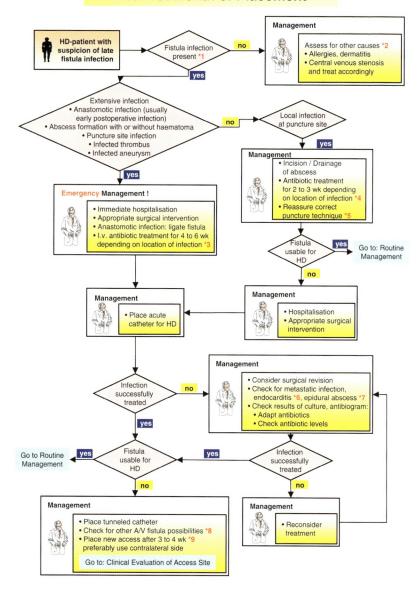

Management of Autogenous A/V Fistula Infection after 1st Month of Placement

*1 Fistula infection present
- Clinical signs of infection are tenderness, erythema, warmth, induration, local serous or purulent discharge and skin ulcers. However, even in the absence of these clinical signs, infection may be present, especially in cases of unexplained sepsis, leukocytosis or fever.
- If fistula infection is suspected, a re-evaluation of precautionary measures to prevent infections, e.g. the correct puncture technique (see ***5** below) and treatment of nasal S. aureus carriers, must be performed (see Algorithm "Routine Management of A/V Fistula and Graft", ***8**).

*2 Assess for other causes
- It is important to distinguish infection from skin changes due to allergic dermatitis, venous hypertension, or inflammation secondary to thrombosis. Unfortunately, fistula Infection can present without fever, high leukocyte count or local signs of infection such as redness, warmth or purulent discharge.
- If laboratory parameters such as elevated CRP suggest an infection, other sources of infection, e.g. infection of a diabetic foot, should also be excluded.

*3 Antibiotic treatment up to 6 weeks
- Extensive A/V fistula infection should be treated like subacute bacterial endocarditis with six weeks of parenteral antibiotics. Excision of the fistula is only necessary in case of infected thrombi and septic emboli[1]. For details of treatment see Appendix "Antibiotic Treatment".

*4 Antibiotic treatment for 2 to 3 weeks
- Localised puncture site infections should be treated with antibiotics for at least two weeks in the absence of fever and bacteraemia, and at least for four weeks in presence of fever and / or bacteraemia[1].

*5 Check correct puncture technique
- Infection of A/V fistulas after the first month of placement is usually due to a violation in the aseptic procedure of vascular access handling. Aseptic handling procedure of the vascular access must be completely reconsidered. The protocol for A/V fistula needling must be revised in concert with a hygienist and/or the local infection control committee. Nursing staff and other care providers must be briefed and trained to strictly apply established protocols. Hygienic rules of how to prepare the patient must be reconsidered. Washing and cleaning procedures of the patient's hands and arms must be reinforced. Skin disinfection must be adapted and the choice of the disinfecting agent and the application time on the skin must be considered.
- Patients at risk, such as chronic carriers of pathogenic bacteria, patients with stomata or with infectious urological disorders must be identified and treated accordingly. Nursing staff must reinforce the aseptic conditions of A/V fistula needling. Hand washing with disinfecting soap is required. The use of sterile gloves, mask and gown is highly desirable during the needling procedure and the use of sterile drape to isolate the skin area for needling, is advised in high risk patients, although expensive and time-consuming.
- Similarly, aseptic technique should be used for the removal of needles and while applying pressure to the puncture sites for haemostasis post dialysis (see Appendix: "Aseptic techniques").

Management of Autogenous A/V Fistula Infection after 1st Month of Placement

- Nursing staff should be examined for nasal carriage of S. aureus, and bacteria should be eradicated with mupirocin ointment.

*6 Endocarditis
- Endocarditits may occur in up to 12 percent of bacteraemia in dialysis patients. As the mortality is high (patient survival after 30 days was only 71 %), it has been proposed that transoesophageal echocardiography should always be performed to exclude endocarditis in patients with positive blood cultures[2].

*7 Epidural abscess
- Bacteraemia might also lead to epidural abscesses. Therefore epidural abscess should be excluded in all patients with recently treated or ongoing bacteraemia and severe back pain[3, 4].

*8 Check for other A/V fistula possibilities
- In the case of an infected forearm A/V fistula, the construction of a new access at the elbow level ought to be considered. The decision can be facilitated substantially by ultrasonographic investigations to exclude perivascular infectious material and/or haematoma. In addition, the status of the venous segment selected for a new A/V anastomosis can be reliably defined. If the infection is located in the region of the elbow, there will be only a limited number of alternatives to create another A/V fistula.
- In any case of severe infection and delayed healing, the contralateral arm should be considered for the construction of a new vascular access since it may be much simpler to create a new access there than to perform major repair surgery of the formerly infected arm. In these situations, native A/V fistulas have absolute priority. In the presence of any infection, insertion of graft material has to be avoided.

*9 Place new access after 3 to 4 weeks
- After complete resolution of local and systemic signs of infection, a new access can be constructed. The risk of re-infection is very low, when no prosthetic material is used[5, 6, 7]. A new A/V fistula can be created in the same arm, if there are suitable vessels remaining. If this is not the case, the other arm must be used. A new autogenous A/V fistula should, of course, be preferred to a graft.

References see p. 146

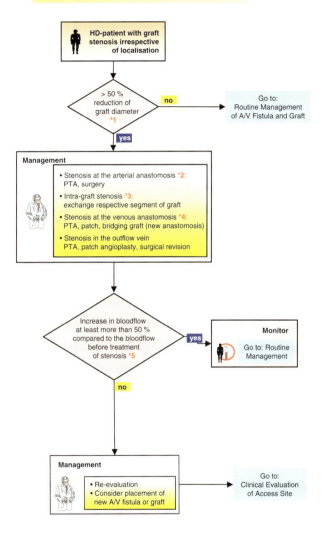

Management of Graft Stenosis

***1 More than 50 % reduction of graft diameter**
- A reduction of > 50 % of the lumen diameter in association with haemodynamic change is recommended as the triggering point for treatment of stenosis[1].
- The impact of the stenosis is more obvious in prescribed blood flows as high as 500 ml/min than in 200 ml/min. The stenosis can lead to a reduction in the adequacy of the dialysis therapy[2]. The progression of the narrowing is quite different in individual patients and, therefore, repeated measurements are necessary to decide whether and how the stenosis should be treated. Multiple stenoses and longer stenoses are probably better treated surgically.

***2 Stenosis at the arterial anastomosis**
- Like in A/V fistulas, most arterial inflow stenoses can successfully be treated by angioplasty.
- Stenosis of the arterial anastomosis itself can be dilated, if only the afferent artery and the graft at the anastomosis is affected but the efferent artery is not stenosed.
- If there is an additional stenosis of the efferent artery, angioplasty of the anastomosis alone will enhance graft flow with the risk of peripheral ischaemia due to reduced peripheral arterial perfusion. In these patients, either dilatation of the efferent artery by interventional radiology or through surgical revision of the anastomosis, may resolve the problem.

***3 Intra-graft stenosis**
- Intra-graft (or mid-graft) stenoses are found in the cannulation segment of access grafts which have been in use for at least some months. They result from excessive in-growth of fibrous tissue through puncture holes. These stenoses can be treated by percutaneous transluminal angioplasty (PTA)[3], graft curettage[4], and segmental graft replacement.
- Replacing the damaged graft segment is not only the most straight-forward but also the most durable means to restore or maintain graft patency[5]. When only part of the cannulation segment is replaced (the remaining can be treated by curettage or intraoperative PTA if necessary), the access can be used for further haemodialysis without the need of a central venous catheter.
- When re-stenosis occurs in a non-exchanged part of the graft, this can be replaced after healing of the new segment (i.e. after two weeks), again without the need for central venous access.

***4 Stenosis at the venous anastomosis**
- The most frequent cause for access graft dysfunction and thrombosis is venous anastomotic stenosis[3,6,7]. As access grafts should be implanted only in patients with exhausted peripheral veins, vein saving procedures like PTA or patch angioplasty should be preferred to graft extensions to more central vein segments, although the latter may provide superior patency rates[8,9].
- When PTA repeatedly fails, additional stent implantation can be considered[10,11]. When stent or a patch fail, graft extension is still possible. This staged application of different therapeutic options is very likely to enhance cumulative graft function to a greater extent than primary use of the "best" option.
- When the interval between the recurrence of stenosis becomes shorter, surgery should be considered.
- Frequent graft occlusion can occur in severely hypotensive patients, in certain

types of thrombophilia, and in subclinical graft infections. These conditions have to be excluded if no or mild stenosis (< 50 %) is found at graft thrombectomy.

*5 Flow at least plus > 50 % of baseline
- After successful percutaneous transluminal angioplasty (PTA) the access blood flow (Q_a) usually increases almost twofold, but in half of the grafts the blood flow decreases to baseline within three months[12]. There is no correlation between the change in blood flow and the residual stenosis[13, 14]. In 20 – 30 % of the grafts, PTA does not increase blood flow to more than 600 ml/min, indicating insufficient dilatation with an undersized balloon, immediate recurrence of stenosis, or the existence of unidentified and not corrected stenosis either more centrally or at the arterial inflow.
- Long-term outcomes did not correlate with angiographic results, but with Qa values before PTA and the increase in Qa due to the procedure[14]. However, it may be argued, that the dilatation has not been sufficient in these grafts.

References see p. 146

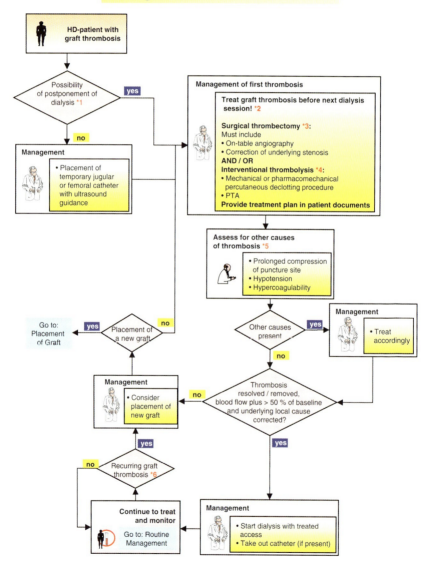

Management of Graft Thrombosis

*1 Postpone dialysis whenever possible
- As in patients with native A/V fistulas, postponement of dialysis may be possible in patients who are not expected to develop pulmonary oedema. Increase of body weight since the last dialysis session will indicate the amount of excess fluid retained. Furthermore, the patients must not show symptoms of uraemia, and the potassium level must not exceed 5.6 mmol/l.

*2 Treat graft thrombosis before next dialysis session
- Graft thrombosis should be treated without unnecessary delay and within 48 hours whenever possible. Early declotting allows for immediate use of the access without the need for central venous access. There is always a compact "arterial plug" present. Mature thrombi older than five days often are fixed to the vessel wall beyond the venous anastomosis, making surgical extraction more difficult. This is less of a problem for the interventional radiologist.
- Central venous catheters should be avoided whenever possible.

*3 Surgical thrombectomy
- Surgical thrombectomy is performed with a embolectomy catheter. A longitudinal incision at the venous anastomosis can be performed with the option of patch plasty. Alternatively an oblique incision of the graft within a reasonable distance of the venous anastomosis can be performed when intraoperative balloon dilatation of the suspected stenosis or surgical graft extension is planned. On-table completion angiography of the arterial and venous limbs of the graft as well as the central venous outflow is mandatory to exclude persistent thrombi and define the cause of thrombosis if it is not venous outlet stenosis. Identification and simultaneous correction of the underlying stenosis are integral parts of any surgical or interventional declotting procedure[1, 2] (see Algorithm "Management of Graft Stenosis" ***3, *4, *5**).

*4 Interventional thrombolysis
- PTFE graft thrombosis is commonly treated using a range of percutaneous techniques including combinations of thromboaspiration, use of thrombolytic agents such as tissue plasminogen activator (tPA), mechanical thrombectomy and mechanical thrombectomy devices. In one study, success rate was 73 %, with primary patency rates of only 32 % and 26 % at one and three months, respectively[3].
- Comparing different mechanical devices for percutaneous thrombolysis, Smits et al. concluded, that "the treatment of the underlying stenoses was the only predictive value for graft patency"[4], which holds truth, as long as the thrombus is actually removed, although not true for all the techniques used.
- Surgery or interventional radiology? Each centre should choose the technique according to their expertise. Independent of the applied technique it is important to perform:
    a) Thrombolysis or thrombectomy rapidly (within 48 hrs) to avoid the need for a temporary catheter.
    b) Thrombolysis or thrombectomy as an outpatient procedure to decrease costs, whenever possible.
    c) Post-procedural angiography to detect and correct inflow, intra-access or outflow venous stenosis[5]. The latter is present in 85 % of thrombosed grafts.
    d) Post-procedural documentation of residual stenosis and access blood flow.

- Quality indicators of successful thrombolysis / thrombectomy are[6]:
  a) Immediate patency (access usable for next haemodialysis treatment) in 85 % of the cases.
  b) Unassisted patency at three months of at least 40 %.
- Dougherty et al. randomly assigned 80 patients to either surgical thrombectomy with patch plasty or interposition of a graft or to thrombolytic therapy with percutaneous transluminal angioplasty if indicated. No difference in outcome was seen, but thrombolytic therapy with PTA was more expensive than the surgical intervention[1]. This study, however, has been criticised for its design (unblinded), for lacking sufficient information regarding the endovascular techniques used, and for incomplete cost analysis[7].
- Marston et al. compared surgical (n = 56) versus endovascular (n = 59) management of thrombosed grafts. While immediate success rates were high in both groups (83 % and 72 %, respectively), patency rates were significantly higher with surgical intervention than with endovascular intervention (36 % versus 11 % after 6 months)[2]. It was pointed out, however, that the 31 % initial failure rate of the percutaneous approach was especially high in this study when compared to the close to 100 % success rates of many other series. This was possibly due to the lack of preoperative imaging before access creation, explaining the high rate of long outflow stenoses unmasked after declotting[8].
- In contrast, Turmel-Rodrigues et al. found higher patency rates after radiological intervention, with a 6 month primary patency rate of 32 % in thrombosed grafts[9].
- While the DOQI guidelines determined a threshold of 40 % for 1-year primary patency rate after surgical treatment of thrombosed grafts[6], none of the three most recent series reached that goal since rates ranged from 23 to 26 %[1,2,10].
- Bakran and McWilliams in an invited commentary on the radiology versus surgery debate pointed out the dearth of good quality of randomised controlled trials dealing with this subject. In some series both surgery and angioplasty had poor outcome[2,11], whilst others had better outcome for angioplasty[12], and yet others had good results from surgery[13]. Their conclusion was that individual centres should audit their own results and choose the modality that produces the best results for that centre. Inevitably, in some centres this will mean angioplasty but in others surgery[14].
- In their recent meta analysis of randomised, controlled trials, Green et al. compared the results of surgical thrombectomy, mechanical thrombectomy and pharmacomechanical thrombolysis for thrombosed dialysis grafts[15]. They found a clear superiority of surgery over endovascular procedures in terms of technical success and patency rates. No differences in complication rates between the groups were demonstrated.

*5 **Assess for other causes of thrombosis**
- The vast majority of access thromboses are due to graft stenosis (see Algorithm "Management of Graft Stenosis"). Other causes such as post-dialysis hypotension, excessive dehydration, hypercoagulability, trauma, or prolonged compression of puncture site are associated risk factors or triggers that often reveal an underlying stenosis.
- Infection can also cause or be associated with access thrombosis.

*6 Recurring graft thrombosis

- Recurring graft thrombosis can be repeatedly treated by interventional radiology. Mansilla found similar re-occlusion rates after the first, second and third radiological treatment[16]. In cases of frequent or early re-stenosis of the venous graft anastomosis, stent implantation can be considered. Stents do not preclude re-stenosis, but slight over-dilating the stent (not more than 1 or 2 mm, see Appendix 4.1.1. PTA) may postpone clinical appearance of re-stenosis[17].
- Surgery (graft extension) should be considered when stenosis- or thrombosis-free intervals gradually become shorter, or when the stenotic segment gradually becomes longer.
- While old, clotted grafts are a potential source of silent infection[16], they should be removed only in cases of otherwise unexplained septicaemia or obvious sepsis.

References see p. 147

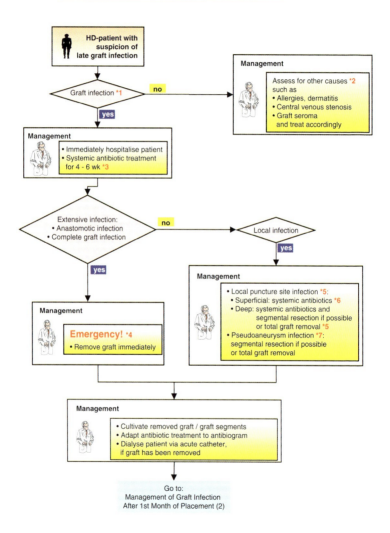

Management of Graft Infection After 1st Month of Placement (1)

*1 Signs of graft infection
- Clinical signs of infection are tenderness, erythema, warmth, induration, local serous or purulent drainage and skin breakdown. However, even in the absence of these clinical signs, infection might be present, especially in cases of unexplained sepsis, leukocytosis or fever of unknown origin.
- Old clotted grafts may be a silent source of infection, which should be investigated by indium scanning since infected grafts show a marked indium uptake[1]. These occult infections of old non-functioning grafts can be a cause of chronic inflammation and resistance to erythropoetin in haemodialysis patients.
- In cases of graft infection, a re-evaluation of precautionary measures to prevent infections, e.g. the correct puncture technique and treatment of nasal S. aureus carriers, must be performed (see Algorithm „Routine Management of A/V Fistula and Graft" ***0**).
- If laboratory parameters, e.g. an elevated CRP, suggest an infection, other sources of infection, e.g. infection of a diabetic foot, should be excluded also.

*2 Assess for other causes
- It is important to distinguish infection from skin changes due to allergic dermatitis, venous hypertension, central stenosis, inflammation or lymph/fluid collections (peri-graft seroma) secondary to the creation of the subcutaneous tunnel.

*3 Systemic antibiotic treatment for 4 - 6 weeks plus surgical intervention
- Treatment of graft infections should always include surgical intervention in combination with systemic antibiotic treatment for 3 – 4 weeks[2, 3]. Only mere superficial infection, which does not involve the graft, may respond to antibiotic therapy alone (see Appendix "Antibiotic Treatment").
- Infection of the graft must be considered in case of suppuration or bleeding from a former needle site. The patient should be hospitalised immediately, blood and wound cultures taken, and systemic antibiotic therapy instituted (see Appendix "Antibiotic Treatment").
After local control of inflammation, resection of the infected graft segment, if possible, or complete graft removal should be performed[4, 5, 6]. In cases of heavy bleeding, urgent surgery is inevitable.

*4 Anastomotic / complete graft infection
- Extensive infections present with purulent discharge, abscess or infected aneurysmal dilatation[2]. They require resection of the total graft and systemic antibiotic therapy in order to prevent bacteraemia, sepsis, haemorrhage and death[3, 6]. In these patients, a delayed tunnelled central venous access should be placed, and the next access should be constructed on the other arm after complete resolution of local and/or systemic signs of infection.

*5 Local puncture site infection
- Localised soft tissue or graft infections after complete healing (after the first month) can occur due to bacterial inoculation during puncture for haemodialysis at a frequency of 5 % per year[4].
- If possible, segmental resection of the infected part should be performed. Otherwise, resection of the complete graft becomes necessary. Conservative excision of the graft has a high recurrence rate and needs close follow-up. Nevertheless, if

segmental graft excision/bypass is performed, several authors recommend leaving some parts of the old graft in place, so that this segment can be used for haemodialysis, thereby avoiding the need for dialysis through a central venous catheter[4, 5].

*6 Superficial infections without graft involvement
- Superficial soft tissue inflammation around a well incorporated graft can be treated with antibiotics alone (see ***3**).

*7 Pseudoaneurysm infection
- Graft pseudo-aneurysms with parietal thrombus are prone to blood-borne or needling-induced infection. There is a high risk of septicaemia and of bleeding due to skin erosion. Treatment consists of antibiotics and surgical segmental graft excision / bypass.

References see p. 148

Management of Graft Infection after 1st Month of Placement (2)

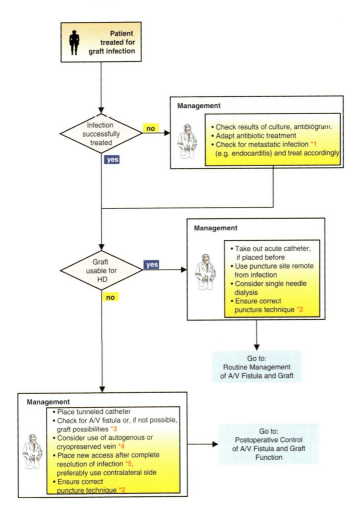

Management of Graft Infection After 1st Month of Placement (2)

***1 Check for metastatic infection**
- Infected grafts can cause metastatic infections, including subdural (epidural) abscesses[1, 2], septic arthritis, osteomyelitis[3] and right and left endocarditits and subsequent septic venous embolization into the lung[4].

***2 Ensure correct puncture technique**
- Puncturing the graft must be performed under aseptic conditions (for details see Appendix chapter "Aseptic techniques").

***3 Check for other access options, A/V fistula / graft**
- Forearm graft infection leading to graft resection leaves the option of creating a native A/V fistula in the ipsilateral upper arm. Usually, cephalic and/or basilic veins proximal to the elbow are dilated due to the presence of the forearm graft. These veins can be evaluated by inspection and palpation and/or duplex imaging. If they are adequate, a brachiocephalic or brachiobasilic A/V fistula in the ipsilateral extremity can be created. In case of inadequate upper arm veins or in case of upper arm graft resection due to infection, the contralateral extremity may be used.
- Preoperative venous mapping is of particular importance in patients with a failed vascular access in order to decide where to place the next A/V fistula, as physical examination has its limitations especially in obese and elderly patients[5]. Thus, duplex ultrasound (see Algorithms "Placement of forearm A/V Fistula") or, in the case of a history of central vein catheterisation, at the site of planned access, venography is indicated.

***4 Consider use of autologous or cryopreserved vein**
- Cryopreserved human femoral veins can be used for creating new accesses, as they are more resistant to infection. There is limited data on the use of cryopreserved femoral vein grafts for difficult haemodialysis access but they have even been placed in the setting of systemic and local infection with good results[6]. Matsura et al. placed 38 cryografts in patients with infection[7]. None of their patients developed graft infections. One year primary and secondary patency were 49 % and 75 %, respectively. Further studies are necessary to define the appropriate role of this graft material.

***5 Place new access after complete resolution of infection**
- After complete resolution of local and systemic signs of infection, a new access can be constructed. In order to reduce the risk of re-infection, prosthetic material should be avoided. Re-infection occurred in 3 out of 9 accesses when a new PTFE graft was created within a mean of three months (range 1 – 10 months)[8].
- A new native A/V fistula using translocated long saphenous vein can be constructed before complete resolution of local and systemic signs of infection. The site of local infection should be avoided.

References see p. 148

Aneurysm

Management of Aneurysms

Patient with access aneurysm

Assessment

Physical examination *1
- Size and growth of aneurysm
- Postaneurysmal stenosis
- Local signs of infection including thrombophlebitis
- Skin quality

- Infection and/or
- Rapid expansion and/or
- Skin damage or
- Threat to skin

yes →

Management:
- Surgical correction *2

no ↓

- Graft pseudo-aneurysm
- Fistula vein aneurysm
- Long segment dilatation of fistula vein

Assessment

Duplex ultrasound for *4:
- Stenosis, pre-/postaneurysm
- Flow reduction
- Thrombus lining wall

Assessment

Duplex ultrasound for:
- Stenosis, junctional *4
- Flow reduction / high flow
- Thrombus lining wall

Presence of:
- Thrombus lining wall
- Postaneurysmal stenosis
- Affection of arterial anastomosis

Presence of:
- Junctional stenosis
- Thrombus lining wall
- High flow

Management:
- Ensure correct needling *3
- Avoid area puncture *3
- Exclude stenosis of venous anastomosis by duplex ultrasound *4
- Surgery: Timely segmental graft replacement before rupture and/or skin damage

Management
- Treat underlying cause accordingly, either surgically or by radiological intervention
- Correction of:
  - Aneurysm at the arteriovenous anastomosis
  - Aneurysm and upstream stenosis
  - Stenosis between aneurysms
  - Long stenosis
  - Postaneurysmatic stenosis

Go to: Routine Management

Management of Aneurysms

*1 Physical examination
- Aneurysms are localised dilatations of vessels. In A/V fistulas aneurysms can be caused by access stenosis, either by pre-stenotic dilation due to increased pressure, or by post-stenotic dilatation due to increased turbulence. Aneurysmal dilatation can also be caused by excessive high flow. Pseudo-aneurysms present as expansile swellings caused by persistent subcutaneous bleeding outside the fistula vein wall or graft. They develop more frequently in grafts than in A/V fistulas and are sometimes the consequence of area puncture with weakening or destruction of the access wall but more often due to poor needling technique, resulting in the need for emergency surgical repair.
- Graft pseudo-aneurysms sometimes develop at the anastomosis due to dehiscence of the suture line.
- Remodelling of the vein due to increased flow leads to a dilatation of the vein. The diagnosis "aneurysm" refers to dilated segments, whose diameter exceeds 1.5 to 2-fold the diameter of the non-dilated access.
- There is no data correlating the diameter of the aneurysm with the frequency of complications, e.g. thrombosis, infection, skin necrosis and rupture. Thus, the indication for intervention must be made on clinical grounds. In general surgical intervention is required in any aneurysm which is rapidly expanding, endangering the viability of the overlying skin, or shows signs of infection, which is especially frequent with pseudo-aneurysms.

*2 Surgical correction
- Aneurysms of A/V fistulas are treated by resection of the aneurysmal segment. Sometimes an end-to-end anastomosis is possible, but often the resected segment must be bridged by a graft. Alternatively a new arterio-venous anastomosis may be created using the vein proximal to the aneurysm.
- In grafts there are two kinds of aneurysms: single, large, symptomatic aneurysms and multiple aneurysms along the entire graft. The former might be treated by resection of the dilated part and interposition of a new graft allowing the remaining segments of the old graft to be used for dialysis. In cases of multiple aneurysms, a long piece of PTFE may be used to replace the aneurysmal graft, but using the arterial and venous anastomoses of the old graft[1].

*3 Ensure correct needling / Avoid area puncture
- Repeated needling of the same area (area puncture) must be avoided as it may result in pseudo-aneurysm formation in a graft. Puncturing a pseudo-aneurysm may lead to rupture of the aneurysm and bleeding. Expanding pseudo-aneurysms must be treated by early and adequate surgical reconstruction of the access, additional skin flap procedure if necessary, and eventual treatment of the down-flow stenosis with which it is frequently associated.

*4 Duplex ultrasound (of aneurysms)
- Aneurysms should be investigated by duplex ultrasound to distinguish between pseudo and true aneurysms, to precisely localise them, measure access blood flow, search for stenosis with either pre- or post-stenotic aneurysm as well as parietal thrombi in the aneurysm.

References see p. 149

Management of High Flow in A/V Fistula and Graft

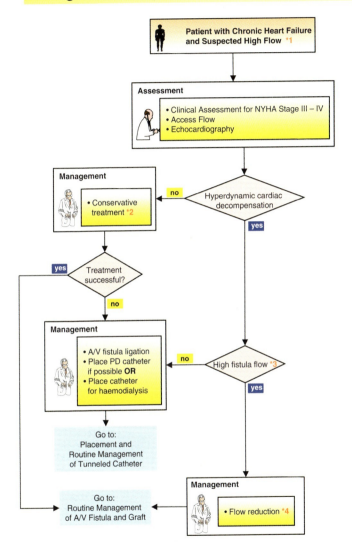

Management of High Flow in A/V Fistula and Graft

*1 Suspected high flow
- Cases of long-term high flow have been published as complications of both distal and proximal A/V fistulas but it is more important and occurs earlier in upper arm fistulas[1-6]. While Murphy et al. reported one case of cardiac failure in 74 brachiobasilic A/V fistulas[7], Ono et al. reported one case of congestive heart failure out of four axillary artery to contralateral axillary vein bridge grafts[8].
- As the aetiology of cardiac failure in dialysis patients is complex (including anaemia, fluid overload, uncontrolled hypertension, intrinsic cardiac disease) the diagnosis of high-output cardiac failure may be overlooked for some time[5].
- The creation of an A/V fistula, however, does not necessarily lead to a significant increase in cardiac load after fistula maturation[1, 9].

*2 Conservative treatment
- Conservative treatment should include control of body weight, modest exercise, diet and medical treatment (ACE inhibitors, AT1-receptor antagonists, β-blockers, diuretics, digitalis etc.), as recommended by current guidelines.

*3 High fistula flow
- For many years, there was no consensus among physicians about the upper limit of normal access flow[2]. When access flow is greater than 1000-1500 ml/min[1] or flow/cardiac output ratio > 20 %[10], then cardiac failure may result.
- Depending on the condition of the patient, cardiac failure may occur at different access flow rates. Extreme flow rates of up to 19.4 l/min have been described in a 27-year old male patient in superb physical condition[6]. Most patients will show cardiac failure with lower access flows.

*4 Flow reduction
- In flow reduction by banding or interposition grafting may be an option to limit bloodflow through the A/V fistula. The results of these procedures, however, are usually disappointing due to insufficient flow reduction or uncontrolled flow increase after the operation.
- More appropriate measures are the following:
  - In the case of a distal radio-cephalic A/V fistula, ligation of the radial artery proximally to the anastomosis results in significant flow reduction, because afterwards the A/V fistula is fed only by the ulnar artery via the palmar arch[11].
  - In the case of an elbow A/V fistula (brachiocephalic or brachiobasilic), moving the arterial anastomosis distally will cause a flow reduction of about 50 %[12]. The anastomosis of vein or graft to the brachial artery is ligated, and a vein or graft is inserted connecting the proximal or distal radial or ulnar artery with the old access.
  - Radial artery transposition is an alternative method to reduce excessive high flow in proximal fistulas. Following ligation of the brachiocephalic or brachiobasilic access anastomosis, the radial artery is transected and dissected in the forearm, and then anastomosed to the access vein at the elbow. Mean flow reduction is 65 %[12].
  - It is obvious that preoperative and postoperative access flow measurements are mandatory in patients with flow reducing operations.

References see p. 149

Ischaemia (1)

Management of Ischaemia (1)

Patient with symptoms of ischaemia in access arm

Assessment
- **Medical history *1**
- **Clinical staging of ischaemia *2**
  - Skin: - temperature and colour
    - ulceration, acral necrosis
  - Pain: - on exercise
    - during haemodialysis
    - rest pain

- Loss of motion
- Reduction in sensation

yes → **Management**: **Emergency!** Surgical intervention *3

no ↓

- Stage I: cold hand
- Stage II: pain on exertion, elevation, during dialysis
  - Graft *6
  - A/V fistula *7
- Stage III: rest pain
- Stage IV: acral necrosis

Monitor ischaemia
"Wait and see" *4, check for deterioration *5

Ischaemia aggravating — no / yes

Assessment
- (Doppler) wrist brachial pressure index *8
- Digital arterial pressure *8
- Access compression: hyperaemia *8
- Duplex ultrasound: retrograde inflow into access
- Imaging *9: transfemoral arteriovenography including complete arterial inflow and peripheral arteries after compression of access

- Peripheral arterial disease → Go to: Management of Ischaemia (2)
- Central arterial disease → **Management**: Interventional or surgical correction *11

Ischaemia successfully treated — yes → Go to: Routine Management of A/V Fistula and Graft
— no → Reassess imaging for peripheral arterial disease

Management of Ischaemia (1)

*1 Medical history
- Some patients are at increased risk of developing hand ischaemia after creation of a vascular access, particularly when the brachial artery is the inflow vessel to the fistula. Risk factors are repeated access surgery on the same extremity, older age, small size of the brachial artery, diabetes and peripheral vascular disease[1]. Patients are often symptomatic at the moment the access has been created[1] and, therefore, they should be closely monitored during the first 24 hours after access creation.

*2 Clinical staging of ischaemia
- Clinical signs and symptoms of steal syndrome do not differ from those of leg ischaemia. Therefore, it can be classified according to Fontaine's classification Stage I, a reduced wrist-brachial pressure index, with coldness of the hand and discolouration (pale or bluish) may be noticed.
Stage II, intermittent pain during haemodialysis[2], exertion or arm elevation occurs.
Stage III, ischaemic rest pain develops.
Stage IV, ulceration and necrosis with or without rest pain develops.
- Symptomatic steal is associated with reduced wrist-to-brachial blood pressure index (< 0.6) as measured by digital photoplethysmography, with blood pressure cuff and Doppler probe, or by transcutaneous pO_2 measurement[3]. The cuff and Doppler method can be done in the clinic, on the ward or in the operating theatre.
- In the differential diagnosis of rest pain, ischaemic monomelic neuropathy, uraemic or diabetic neuropathy, secondary hyperparathyroidism, carpal tunnel syndrome and venous hypertension with ulcerative skin changes have to be considered[4, 5].

*3 Surgical intervention
- Ischaemia can occur at any time, directly after the creation of a vascular access or much later. Irreversible damage can be caused to nerves within hours due to severe ischaemia, labelled ischaemic monomelic neuropathy. Therefore, patients with significantly impaired nerve function, motor or sensory, must be treated as an emergency.

*4 "Wait and see"
- Stage I and II steal syndrome in both A/V fistulas and grafts can be closely observed and treated conservatively (wearing gloves).

*5 Check for deterioration
- Especially in A/V fistulas already at stage I of ischaemia, close clinical monitoring must be performed. Due to the tendency of flow to increase over time, stage I disease may deteriorate. Monitoring consists of regularly asking the patient about symptoms of exertional or rest pain, increasing coldness and colour changes of the hand, examining the hand for development of ischaemic lesions, and assessing the wrist brachial pressure index.
- The onset of vascular steal can be delayed up to several months after surgery[6].

*6 Access graft
- Contrary to the course of steal syndrome in A/V fistulas (see ***7**), grafts even in stage II can improve, when venous anastomotic stenosis begins to reduce flow. These patients must be monitored not only for symptoms of their steal syndrome but also for access flow. When deterioration of graft function necessitates therapy,

simultaneous treatment of steal syndrome is advised to prevent severe post-operative or post-interventional ischaemia.

*7 A/V fistula
- Once an A/V fistula causes stage II steal syndrome, further diagnostic assessment is indicated, and timely correction of steal syndrome should be done before progression to stage III or IV disease if objective assessment indicates reduction in perfusion pressure in the hand.

*8 Access compression and duplex ultrasound
- Steal syndrome occurs when there is diastolic retrograde inflow from the distal artery into the A/V fistula or graft. This phenomenon can easily be demonstrated by colour-coded duplex-sonography. Digital compression of the access without compression of the artery but complete blockade of access flow will return distal arterial flow direction to normal, thus improving peripheral circulation and usually return of distal pulses can be observed. Reactive hyperaemia is seen within seconds and can be detected by pulse oximetry, continuous transcutaneous pO_2 ($tcpO_2$) measurement, increase in the wrist brachial pressure index or digital photoplethysmography [3, 7, 8].

*9 Imaging: Upper limb arteriography
- Every patient with steal syndrome has to undergo thorough examination of his or her respective arm's complete arterial tree[1, 5]. After introducing an angiography catheter from the femoral or from the ipsilateral brachial artery via the Seldinger technique, all the arteries of the upper limb must be opacified from the ostium of the subclavian artery to the digital arteries. Due to the severely impaired arterial outflow, peripheral arteries can be sufficiently visualised (in most patients) only after digital compression of the access.

*10 Nerve conduction
- Ischaemic Monomelic Neuropathy (IMN). IMN leads to almost irreversible development of severe sensorimotor dysfunction distal to the arteriovenous anastomosis, sometimes without obvious tissue loss. IMN is thought to occur due to transient nerve ischaemia insufficient to cause tissue necrosis but resulting in severe nerve injury in susceptible patients (e.g. diabetics)[4].
- Waiting for the results of detailed nerve conduction studies must not lead to postponement of treatment in cases with unequivocal clinical signs and symptoms of IMN. Very urgent closure of the arteriovenous anastomosis is considered by many as the only way to avoid significant loss of sensorimotor function.

*11 Interventional or surgical correction
- Central arterial stenoses (subclavian, axillary, brachial artery) proximal to the access can be dilated via the transfemoral route or in a retrograde fashion after cannulation of the access or of the brachial artery[5, 7, 9, 10]. The high arteriovenous flow seems to reduce the frequency of re-stenose[9]. If complete arterial occlusion cannot be reopened interventionally, standard vascular surgical bypass must be performed.

References see p. 150

Management of Ischaemia (2)

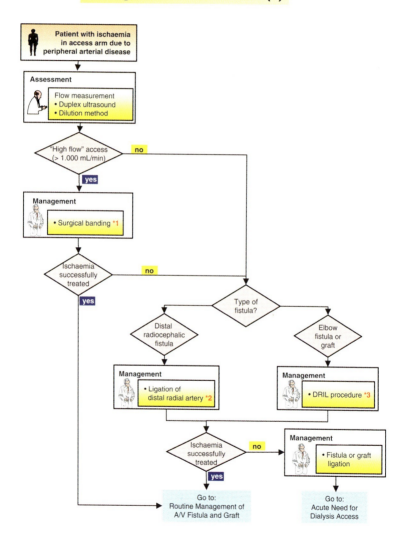

Management of Ischaemia (2)

*1 Surgical banding
- Surgical banding of the access is usually performed close to the arterial anastomosis. A/V fistulas can be banded with non-absorbable sutures, a small calibre interposition graft, or by narrowing the vein with a tight Dacron or PTFE cuff. In prosthetic access, interposition of a short tapered graft segment has been suggested. All these procedures create a reduction in blood flow up the fistula and steal syndrome will disappear after a sufficient reduction in fistula blood flow or cessation of reversal of diastolic retrograde inflow from the distal brachial artery. This can be achieved only when access resistance at least approaches the level of peripheral arterial resistance. Sufficient surgical banding thus means suturing a high grade anastomotic stenosis with the risk of insufficient flow or even access thrombosis[1, 2]. Therefore, banding should be attempted only with intraoperative monitoring of access flow as well as peripheral circulation (pulse oximetry, continuous transcutaneous pO_2 ($tcpO_2$) measurement, digital photoplethysmography, pulse volume recordings or Doppler wrist/brachial pressure index measurement[3, 4]).
- Despite subtle technique, access banding results in high rates of thrombosis or recurring steal[1].
- See also Algorithm: "Management of high flow in A/V fistula and grafts".

*2 Ligation of distal radial artery
- The easiest way to block retrograde arterial inflow into a distal access at the wrist is to ligate (or embolise) the artery distally to the anastomosis. In radio-cephalic (or ulnar-basilic) fistulae, the effect can be simulated by digital compression of the respective artery at the wrist below the anastomosis. In 1971, Bussell et al. demonstrated an increase in pulse amplitude of the thumb averaging 80 % in compressing the radial artery distal to the anastomosis, thus impairing retrograde inflow[5]. By compressing the ulnar artery, a 90 % reduction in pulse amplitude of the thumb was seen.
- Before interventional embolisation of the artery, temporary balloon blockade can serve the same purpose. Pulse oximetry, continuous transcutaneous pO_2 ($tcpO_2$) measurement or digital photoplethysmography prior to and after definitive treatment are helpful in quantifying the problem and assessment of the improvement in hand circulation[6].

*3 DRIL procedure
- Arterial ligation distal to the A/V fistula can also be performed successfully in elbow fistulas to treat steal syndrome. Ligation of the brachial artery, however, was felt to enhance the risk of forearm ischaemia. Therefore **D**istal **R**evascularisation was added to **I**nterval **L**igation of the artery. In this so-called DRIL procedure, the artery is ligated distally to the access anastomosis, and a vein bypass from proximal to the anastomosis to distal to the ligation is inserted. It is recommended that construction of the proximal anastomosis should be a reasonable distance (> 5 cm) proximal to the access to prevent diastolic retrograde flow, and thereby recurrence of steal syndrome, within the bypass. Results of DRIL procedure appear reasonable although only a few centres have reported long-term results[1, 7].

*4 **Distal extension of the access**
  - Another alternative which does not involve ligation of a normal brachial artery is to take down the fistula at the anastomosis, thereby reconstituting the brachial artery flow and then using a separate segment of vein to extend the fistula vein onto the proximal or distal radial or ulnar artery. This allows fistula inflow from one forearm artery whilst still allowing distal flow down the other. This has not been published in a series but has been effective in a clinical practice.

*5 **Closure of the access**
  - Closure of the access is often the only reasonable way to limit severe distal necrotic lesions, especially in cases of major arterial calcification and in patients with significant surgical risk factors. When abandoning the access and creating a new one on the other arm, the high risk of steal syndrome in that extremity must be borne in mind. Some of these patients therefore are candidates for permanent central venous haemodialysis access.

References see p. 150

Central Venous Obstruction (1)

Management of Central Venous Obstruction (1)

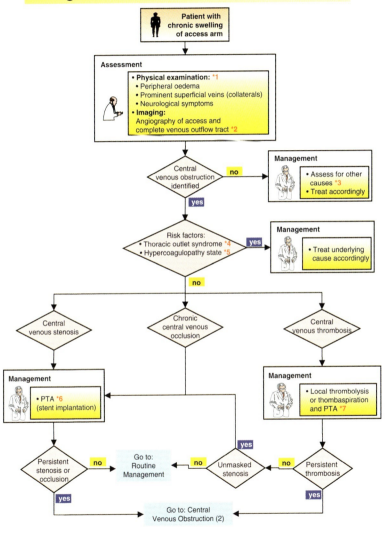

Management of Central Venous Obstruction (1)

*1 Physical examination
- Chronic swelling of the access arm is the most important clinical sign of central venous stenosis[1, 2]. The superficial veins may become prominent (collaterals), and pain and paraesthesia may occur.
- Central venous lesions have to be treated only in cases of clinically significant impairing arm swelling, troublesome pain or if they lead to inadequate haemodialysis. Limited oedema or high venous pressure without consequences on the quality of dialysis are acceptable.

*2 Imaging: Angiography of access and complete venous outflow tract
- Only the lateral part of the subclavian vein can be examined ultrasonographically. To completely visualise all mediastinal veins, venography (using DSA technique) is needed[3, 4]. This can be achieved as arterio-venography via a transfemoral (see Algorithm "Management of Ischaemia (1)", ***9**) or a transbrachial approach, if the arterial access anastomosis is at or distal to the elbow region and arm swelling does not preclude arterial puncture, or, preferably, after direct puncture of the access[5, 6, 7].

*3 Assess for other causes
- In patients without a history of central venous catheterisation, extrinsic compression of mediastinal veins (lymphoma, goitre, thoracic aortic aneurysm, mediastinal fibrosis) should be considered. Plain X-rays and/or computed tomography may be helpful for differential diagnosis. If treatment of the underlying disease is not possible or fails to resolve arm swelling, PTA with stent insertion is indicated[8].
- Chronic uni- or bilateral arm swelling can occur secondarily to extensive axillary or mediastinal lymphatic destruction (post-surgery or post-radiation, primary or metastatic lymphoma, primary mediastinal fibrosis). In some cases, such as lymphoma, treatment of the underlying disease will improve arm swelling.
- If venous stenosis or occlusion is excluded, then access ligation may not have any effect on oedema and hence the fistula may be kept unless, as stated above, it cannot be needled or is causing other symptoms.

*4 Thoracic outlet syndrome
- Axillary-subclavian vein thrombosis may be caused by costoclavicular compression, the so called thoracic outlet syndrome. In order to prevent rethrombosis, transaxillary resection of the first rib should be performed[10]. A relatively infrequent complication is the thrombosis of the subclavian vein of uncertain aetiology. Thrombolysis with urokinase infusion is successful in most cases, otherwise thrombectomy may be performed[9, 10].

*5 Hypercoagulopathy
- Such a condition can be due to reduced levels of protein C and S and factor X or hyperfibrinogenaemia.

*6 PTA (stent implantation)
- Since the late 1980's, several studies of patients treated with PTA alone have been published. Patency rates of 7 % to 12 %[11, 12] at one year were disappointing. Stent implantation has clearly been shown to improve primary one year patency rates to 56 – 76 %[2, 8, 11, 13, 14]. These figures do not differ significantly from those of surgical intervention, where primary one year patency rates between 80 % and 86 %[1, 2, 11, 14] have been reported.

- Due to the relative invasiveness of surgery for central venous obstructions (see Algorithm "Management of Central Venous Obstruction (2)"), the less invasive interventional therapy, PTA with or without stent implantation, is recommended as first-line treatment[14, 15].
- Stent placement should avoid overlapping the ostium of a patent internal jugular vein to achieve a safe and sufficient result, if possible, since this latter vein is essential for future placement of central catheters. Similarly, a stent placed in the brachio-cephalic trunk must not overlap the ostium of the contralateral trunk, otherwise contralateral stenosis may be produced and preclude future use of the contralateral limb for fistula creation[16].

*7 **Local thrombolysis or thrombaspiration**
- Little data is available on the use of thrombolytic agents in central vein thrombosis in dialysis patients although successful thrombolysis has been described in cancer patients treated with thrombolytic agents and PTA[17, 18, 19].

References see p. 151

Management of Central Venous Obstruction (2)

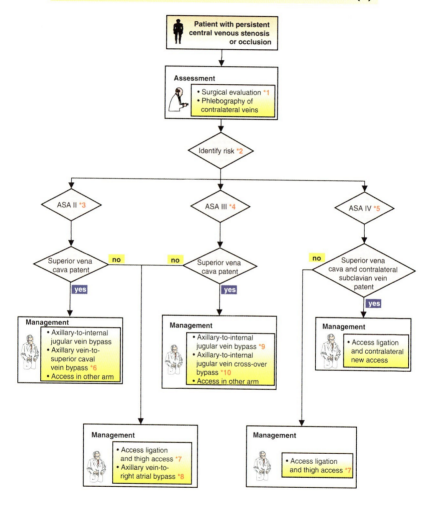

Management of Central Venous Obstruction (2)

*1 Surgical evaluation
- When interventional treatment of central venous obstruction is impossible or fails (in approximately 30 % of cases), thorough assessment of the patient is necessary to define the most effective surgical method to guarantee long-term vascular access for haemodialysis[1]. Surgical evaluation has to focus on the general risk (in terms of the ASA Physical Status Classification System, see this algorithm, ***2**) and life expectancy as well as on the patient's vascular pathology.
- All angiograms have to be re-evaluated. If an ipsilateral surgical bypass is impossible due to brachiocephalic vein obstruction, additional venography of the contralateral arm should be performed to assess whether a new peripheral access can be performed on that arm or a cross-over bypass graft inserted[2, 3, 4].
- In case of bilateral obstruction of mediastinal veins, including the superior vena cava, colour-coded duplex-ultrasonography of ilio-caval veins is indicated in the planning of arterio-venous thigh access.

*2 Identify risk
- The American Society of Anesthesiologists (ASA) has proposed a classification system for risk stratification of surgical patients. It is based on clinical and laboratory findings and has been shown to be one of the best indicators for perioperative morbidity and mortality in a variety of clinical settings. Patients are classified into six groups:
  ASA I: A normal healthy patient
  ASA II: A patient with mild systemic disease
  ASA III A patient with severe systemic disease
  ASA IV: A patient with severe systemic disease that is a constant threat to life
  ASA V: A moribund patient who is not expected to survive without the operation
  ASA VI: A declared brain-dead patient whose organs are being removed for donor purposes.
- Using this definition, patients on chronic renal replacement therapy have to be classified as ASA III or ASA IV. Otherwise healthy patients in the pre-dialysis state (end-stage renal disease or end-stage chronic allograft rejection) with only mild symptoms may be classified as ASA II.

*3 ASA II
- In those rare ASA II patients, with relatively low operative morbidity/mortality and relatively high life expectancy on chronic haemodialysis, every effort should be made to save a functioning access and preserve the contralateral arm for later accesses.
- When only the subclavian vein is occluded, a veno-venous bypass to the ipsilateral internal jugular vein can be performed[2, 5]. When the brachiocephalic vein is occluded, cephalic or axillary vein-to-superior vena cava bypass can be considered even if the contralateral central arm veins are open. However, it is questionable, whether such invasive surgery is justified whilst other more simple peripheral access is possible in the contralateral limb. In patients with chronic occlusion of the superior vena cava, cephalic or axillary vein-to-right atrial bypass have been performed (see this algorithm, ***10**) in order to postpone the need for thigh access (see this algorithm, ***6**) with its consequent risk of losing the last venous territory.

*4 **ASA III**
   - Due to the higher operative risk in ASA III patients, median sternotomy or right thoracotomy for caval or atrial anastomosis should be avoided. When only the subclavian vein is occluded, a veno-venous bypass to the ipsilateral internal jugular vein should be performed[2, 5]. In cases of occlusion of the brachiocephalic vein, cross-over bypass to the contralateral internal jugular vein can be considered[2, 6], although bearing in mind that a peripheral new access in the other arm is likely to be more durable than extra-anatomic veno-venous bypass. Cross-over bypass to a patent axillary vein (with the risk of subsequent stenosis of the vein) has to be avoided, as long as peripheral access on the contralateral arm is possible[4]. Contralateral central arm veins have to be spared until ipsilateral access is no longer possible.

*5 **ASA IV**
   - In patients with high operative risk and reduced life expectancy (ASA IV), ligation of the access is an effective option to treat disabling arm swelling. Creation of a new access in the other arm or thigh should be performed prior to ligation of the fistula in the swollen arm in order to have a matured access at the time of abandonment of the old one.

*6 **Axillary-to-superior caval vein bypass**
   - In case of thrombosis of the subclavian and jugular vein, a bypass from the axillary to the superior caval vein is possible but requires thoracotomy. This should only be performed it there is no other option elsewhere.

*7 **Access ligation and thigh access**
   - For details see "Placement of Graft" ***9.**

*8 **Axillary vein-to-right atrial bypass**
   - There are only a few case reports in the literature of axillary vein-to-right atrial bypass in haemodialysis patients with complete occlusion of the superior vena cava. Patency rates published are better than those for central venous bypasses in non-haemodialysis patients. It is believed that the high flow rates provided by the arterio-venous accesses prevent thrombus formation in veno-venous bypasses[8, 9].
   - In case of superior vena cava occlusion and no other possibility of creating a peripheral vascular access, a subclavian artery to right atrium haemodialysis bridge graft has been successfully performed[10].

*9 **Axillary-to-internal jugular vein bypass**
   - Criado et al. successfully performed the axillary-to-internal jugular vein bypass in two patients[11]. As no thoracotomy is required, this procedure is well suitable for ASA III patients.
   - It is also possible to perform a jugular vein transposition onto the subclavian or axillary vein.
   - Axillary vein obstruction can be treated with a brachio-jugular PTFE-graft[5], although long-term outcome is likely to be poor.

*10 **Axillary-to-internal jugular vein cross-over bypass**
   - In the case of thrombosis of the ipsilateral jugular vein, the bypass can be sutured to the contralateral internal jugular vein.

References see p. 152

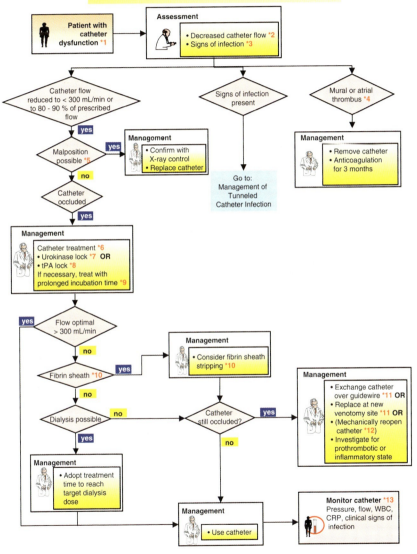

Identification and Management of Tunneled Catheter Complications

*1 Patient with catheter dysfunction
- Haemodialysis vascular access catheters have a significantly higher rate of thrombotic and infectious complications than grafts or native A/V fistulas[1].

*2 Decreased catheter flow
- Permanent tunneled catheters should provide a blood flow of > 300 ml/min to allow for adequate haemodialysis.
- Blood flow should not be measured by roller pump revolution, as this might overestimate blood flow by up to 33 % in the presence of highly negative inflow pressure (– 400 mm Hg)[2].
- Blood flow depends on the size of the catheter and its positioning (see Algorithm "Placement and Routine Management of Permanent Tunneled Catheter" for details) and obstruction / thrombosis of the catheter.
- In cases of insufficient blood flow, differentiation between extrinsic and intrinsic catheter thrombosis should be made. The former may be caused by central vein thrombus, atrial thrombus or mural thrombus, and the latter due to intraluminal thrombus, catheter tip thrombus or fibrin sheath.

*3 Signs of infection
- Catheter-related sepsis is largely based on clinical suspicion. Due to the fact, that dialysis patients frequently present with non-catheter-related infection, it is important to identify the source of any infection in order to avoid unnecessary catheter exchanges[3]. Kite et al. used an endoluminal brush, which allows for sampling of the endoluminal surface of the catheter in situ[4]. The sensitivity and specificity for the diagnosis of catheter-related sepsis was 95 % and 84 %, respectively. However, this procedures is considered by some to be potentially dangerous, due to the risk of disruption of the biofilm.
- Catheter-related infection might also present only with minor signs such as insidious onset of low-grade fever, hypothermia, hypotension, hypoglycaemia, distant abscesses, endocarditis or by symptoms of lethargy and confusion.

*4 Mural or atrial thrombus
- Both types of thrombi are rare but can interfere with catheter function[5].
- It is assumed that the movement of the catheter tip causes damage to the inner wall of the vessel resulting in formation of a thrombus. In such instances, three months of anticoagulation should follow the removal of the catheter[1].

*5 Catheter malposition
- Insufficient blood flow can also be caused by catheter malposition. This can be diagnosed by radiology. In these cases, the catheter should be repositioned or exchanged over a guidewire, the correct positioning should be confirmed by X-ray.

*6 Poor catheter blood flow
- In case of reduced catheter flow or obstruction, fibrinolytic agents like urokinase and tissue plasminogen activator (tPA) can be injected into the catheter ("locking" the catheter) for 30 minutes in the predialysis period, locking the catheter for 24 hours between dialysis sessions or by infusion of the agent for 2-3 hours during the dialysis session.
- If the dysfunction of the catheter cannot be resolved, catheterogram and/or venography is indicated to identify precisely the cause of the catheter dysfunction.

- Relapsing catheter dysfunction may indicate a prothrombotic state of the patient caused by inflammation, latent infection, hyperfibrinogenaemia, high platelet count or other abnormalities of the coagulation cascade. The underlying cause must be treated accordingly. Oral anticoagulation may maintain patency of the catheter in this situation.

*7 Urokinase lock
- Urokinase lock and urokinase infusion have been successfully used to reopen a catheter or to restore catheter flow[6, 7, 8, 9].
- Catheters presenting with low flow high pressures may be locked for 30 minutes with 10,000 units of urokinase (5,000 units per branch), then, re-aspirated and flushed with saline (see appendix for protocol).
- A second protocol is infusion of 50,000 or 100,000 units of urokinase for 20-30 minutes through each catheter lumen.
- Suhocki et al. described successful restoration of catheter flow to > 300 ml/min in 74 % of the cases using urokinase instillation[10].
- Catheters with persisting low flow and high resistance despite short urokinase lock can be infused for 3 hours continuously with urokinase at 100,000 units per hour (50000 units per lumen). The catheter should then be flushed with saline and flow resistance tested.
- Twardowski compared effectiveness of a urokinase lock to an infusion of urokinase[8]. While the urokinase lock was only partly successful in 21 out of 286 occluded catheters, an infusion of 20-40,000 IU urokinase lead to a partial restoration of blood flow in 10 out of 25 patients. Best results were achieved by infusion of 250,000 IU urokinase over 3 hours during dialysis. If necessary, this procedure was repeated during the following dialysis session. Full restoration of catheter flow was achieved at the first attempt in 132 out of 162 catheters with reduced flow.
- In cases of persistent dysfunction a catheterogram and/or a venography is indicated.
- Occluded catheters may be reopened by a combination of mechanical intervention and fibrinolysis based on a continuous urokinase infusion of 100,000 units per hour during 3 hours.
- Urokinase use is not recommended in all situations, and is no longer prescribable in the United States due to safety concerns[7].

*8 tPA lock
- Recombinant tissue plasminogen activator (tPA) is a safe and very effective fibrinolytic agent to dissolve catheter clots and re-establish adequate blood flow[11, 12, 13, 14, 15]. Efficacy of tPA seems to be superior or at least equivalent to urokinase in reopening catheters. One mg of tPA was seen to be as equally as effective as 36,000 units of urokinase[7].
- tPA can also be used either as a catheter lock or as a continuous infusion. Partial catheter obstruction with low flow and high resistance may be resolved either by a tPA catheter infusion for a short period of 2-3 hours[16] or by a catheter lock for a long duration of an interdialysis period of 24-48 hours)[17]. In the latter case it seems appropriate to have a mixture of tPA and heparin as a locking solution.
- Occluded catheters might be reopened by locking each catheter line with 2mg/2mL of tPA with a dwell time of 2 hours, leading to a 74 % success rate of restoring catheter function. If only partial flow recovery occurs, the procedure may be repeated a second time, increasing the success rate to 90 %[15].

- Little et al. investigated the long-term outcome of catheters treated with tPA to restore adequate blood flow[18]. They found the clinical benefit and cost-effectiveness of treating recurrent catheter malfunction with tPA to be limited, since this only allowed for a median of five to seven additional dialysis sessions.

*9 If necessary, treat with prolonged incubation time
- When catheter treatment is unsuccessful (relapsing dysfunction or persistent occlusion) catheter imaging (catheterogram and venography) is indicated.
- In cases of partial catheter thrombosis or fibrin sheath formation around the catheter tip, a prolonged thrombolysis of the catheter may be attempted (see urokinase ***6** or tPA ***7**).

*10 Fibrin sheath
- A fibrin sheath (also called fibrin sleeve) surrounding the catheter tip requires the prolonged infusion of fibrinolytic agent to dissolve the clot. However, this sheath may not only consist of fibrin alone, but also of a tissue, formed by the migration of small muscle cells into the fibrin layer.
- f thrombolysis is not successful in catheters with fibrin sheaths, fibrin sheath stripping by means of a "snare" catheter, led up from the femoral vein, may be indicated. This procedure has a success rate of 79 %[19, 20]. However, this procedure does not provide a durable benefit, as blood flow rates decreased by the 5th session[21]. No significant difference has been found between fibrin sheath stripping and urokinase infusion[22].
- Suhocki et al. increased mean catheter survival to 12.7 months by using thrombolysis and percutaneous mechanical techniques[10].

*11 Exchanging catheters over guidewire – Replace at new venotomy site
- Persisting dysfunction requires the replacement of the catheter. Depending on the type of catheter, exchange may be performed over a guidewire[23]. However, when a fibrin sheath is the cause of reduced blood flow, this sheath may recur around the new catheter also[1]. In addition, infectious complications may be better prevented by insertion of a new catheter at a new venous site. Therefore, new catheter insertion is preferred by some experts to exchange over a guidewire.

*12 Mechanical method to regain catheter patency
- Catheter brushing is a new therapeutic option to re-open the catheter[24]. Bel'eed et al. temporarily restored blood flow in 3 out of 13 patients[25]. The main advantage is to save time for both patient and care providers[26]. However, the use of such a mechanical device is associated with potentially serious hazards that may be underestimated. These include clot embolism with potential lung injury, bacteraemia, trauma of the host vein, perforation of the superior vena cava, right atrium or the ventricle, arrhythmia, or rupture of the catheter. Catheter brushing must, therefore, be carefully performed only by trained physicians under strict fluoroscopy control.

*13 Monitor catheter
- Catheter exit site should be examined for signs of infection at each haemodialysis session.

References see p. 153

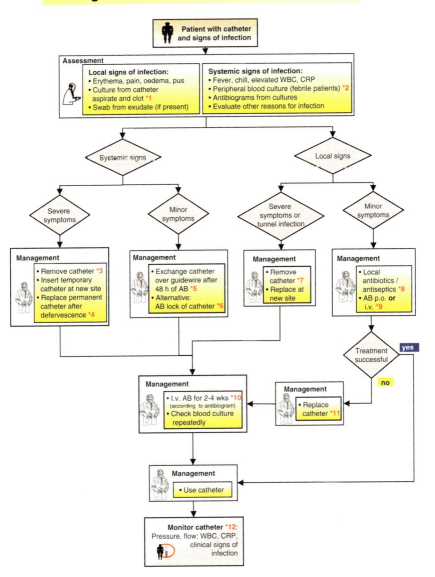

Management of Tunneled Catheter Infection

*1 Culture from catheter aspirate and clot
- Blood from the catheter hub and aspirated clots should be cultured if catheter infection is suspected. Biofilms are frequent in catheters. In over 80 % of biofilms bacterial growth can be proven. The clinical importance, however, is still speculative[1].

*2 Peripheral blood culture
- At least three blood cultures should be taken 10 to 30 minutes apart, one of them should be drawn from the catheter, and the others from peripheral sites.
- Marr et al. defined catheter-related bacteraemia if the same organism could be cultured from the catheter and from a peripheral site or from two peripheral locations[2]. Capdevila et al. described a 94 % sensitivity and a 100 % specificity, if the count of colony-forming units (CFU) was fourfold higher in the blood drawn from the catheter than in simultaneously drawn peripheral blood[3]. A single bacterial count of > 100 CFU/ml from the catheter hub port with an identical organism growing from the peripheral blood specimen is highly suggestive of catheter-related bacteraemia.

*3 Remove catheter
- Immediate removal of the catheter is recommended in case of severe symptoms[4, 5], in clinically unstable patients and in patients who remain symptomatic for more than 36 hours[6].
- Catheter replacement should be delayed (see ***5**)[7, 4, 5].
- After removal of the catheter, the catheter tip should be cultured. The culture result may retrospectively implicate the catheter as the cause of sepsis[8, 9].

*4 Replace after resolution of infection
- A new permanent tunneled catheter should not be placed before resolution of signs and symptoms of bacteraemia and after cultures have been negative for at least two days after cessation of antibiotic therapy[7, 4, 5].

*5 Exchange catheter over a guidewire
- Catheter exchange over a guidewire is a recognised procedure to treat proven or suspected catheter related infection[10, 11, 12, 13]. In one study, exchange over a guidewire led to similar infection-free survival compared with removal and delayed replacement, with fewer procedures for the patient[14].
- However, despite the fact that this option is quoted in the DOQI guidelines, many experts do not recommend such catheter exchange, since this is a way of inducing blood stream infection from a localised source infection (endoluminal catheter infection or track infection). Such procedure may constitute a perfect condition for delayed septic metastasis or endocarditis. Catheter withdrawal and insertion of a new permanent catheter in a different venous site is the recommendable alternative.
- Metastatic endocarditis[15], epidural[16] and psoas abscess[17] have been described in catheter related bacterial infections treated without catheter removal. However, Marr et al. did not find an increased risk of complications in patients where attempts were made to leave the catheter in place[2].
- There is clearly no consensus in the policy regarding how to manage catheter sepsis. Each patient should be managed on his/her merits with risk and benefit considered.

*6 Antibiotic lock of the catheter
- Bacteraemia can also be treated without catheter removal but with an additional antibiotic lock of the catheter after each dialysis session for two weeks. This option has also been proposed by the European Best Practice Guidelines on Haemodialysis[6].
- Infection in permanent Tunneled catheters have been successfully treated with an antibiotic lock of the catheter and systemic antibiotics in 40 out of 79 patients (51 %)[18].
- In an implanted, subcutaneous device for haemodialysis, bacteraemia has been successfully treated with systemic antibiotics and antibiotic lock of the device[19].
- In instances of bacteraemia, antibiotic treatment without antibiotic lock of the catheter and without catheter removal successfully salvaged the catheter in 32 % of the attempts. Marr et al. stated that attempted salvage may not increase the risk of complications[2].

*7 Remove catheter in case of tunnel infection
- Tunnel infections, i.e. infections extending along the tunnel and beyond the cuff in cuffed catheters, are best treated by catheter removal and replacement at a new venotomy site[4, 5].

*8 Local antiseptics
- Isolated exit site infection, i.e. infection distal to the anchoring cuff in cuffed catheters, presenting with redness, exudation and crusts, should be treated conservatively with topical antibiotics or antiseptics (e.g. antibiotic creams such as mupirocin or fucidin or antiseptics such as povidone iodine cream or dressings soaked in hypertonic saline) during the dialysis session[4, 5].
- However, silicone catheters must not be treated with povidone ointment due to possible damage to the catheter.

*9 i.v. antibiotics
- Exit site infections without bacteraemia, which do not respond to therapy with local antibiotics or antiseptics, should be treated with systemic antibiotics for two weeks[6]. Whilst culture results are pending, empirical antibiotic treatment should be initiated and later on adjusted according to the culture and antibiotic sensitivities (see appendix for "Antibiotic Treatment").

*10 Choice of antibiotic treatment
- Immediate antibiotic therapy must be started as soon as infection is suspected and blood samples have been drawn. Initial empirical treatment should take into account the likely bacterial species. Staphylococci are the most prevalent isolates (60 to 90 %) in haemodialysis catheter-related bacteraemia, the relative prevalence of S. aureus and coagulase-negative Staphylococci being equal. Enterococci were found in 11 to 19 % and Gram negative rods have been reported in up to 33 % of the cases[7, 20, 21, 22, 23, 24, 25].
- Systemic antibiotics should be administered for at least two weeks in cases of exit site infection and for at least four weeks following bacteraemia[6]. Blood cultures should be taken repeatedly to monitor effectiveness of the treatment. Antibiotic sensitivities should dictate the antibiotic choice as soon as these are available[4].
- Parenteral antibiotics such as methicillin, cefazolin, vancomycin or teicoplanin are recommended for the initial treatment. When the probability of MRSA is low, vancomycin and teicoplanin should perhaps be reserved as a second-line treatment.

In the United States, however, about 45 – 70 % of the Staphylococci are methicillin resistant (MRSA) which is less of a problem in Europe. MRSA strains with decreased susceptibility to glycopeptides have also been reported, mainly in the dialysis community and may present a challenging problem in the future.
- For details on antibiotic treatment, please refer to appendix chapter "Antibiotic Treatment".

*11 Replacement of catheter in the presence of exit site infection
- The new catheter can be placed through the same venotomy site as the previous one but a new tunnel should be created to avoid the infected site. Alternatively, the catheter should be placed with a new venotomy site, a new tunnel and a new exit site again avoiding the infected skin area[4, 5].

*12 Monitor catheter
- Persistence or recurrence of fever, increase in CRP and white blood cell count or positive blood cultures after catheter removal and antibiotic treatment suggest septic metastasis. Echocardiography or, preferably transoesophageal echocardiography, must be performed to search for endocarditis. Total body scintigraphy with labelled white cells may be helpful in identifying metastatic infection sites, such as in bone and joints.
- Catheter monitoring is mandatory to ensure dialysis efficacy and to prevent catheter-related hazards (see: "Placement of Tunneled Catheter").

References see p. 155

Appendix

1. Diagnostics

1.1. Physical Examination

1.1.1. Examination of Veins
Veins should be dilated during assessment. Therefore, examination should take place in a warm room with the patient feeling comfortable (discomfort and cold lead to vaso-constriction). Examination should include:
- Examination in general
  Inspection of both upper limbs for scars since these may indicate former vascular accesses, other operations, central venous catheter, infection, venous collaterals around the shoulder.
- Examination for size and location of veins
  A blood pressure cuff proximally placed on the arm and inflated to 60 mm Hg or a tourniquet can be used. Clenching and unclenching the hand helps to engorge the veins. The course of the veins should be palpated and they should be distensible up to 2 – 3 mm. The vein should feel soft with no narrowed or thickened areas.
- Examination for venous outflow
  By light percussion on the vein at the wrist, a transmitted wave should be felt at the vein in the elbow region proving the patency of the vein. Before the pressure cuff or tourniquet is released, the arm should be elevated. After releasing the cuff tourniquet, the veins should empty very quickly. Prolonged emptying may suggest venous outflow stenosis.

1.1.2. Examination of Arteries
- Examination for central arterial stenosis
  Blood pressure in both arms should be measured by the Riva-Rocci method. Differences in the systolic blood pressure of > 20 mm Hg, or relative differences of > 10 % (corresponding to an arm/arm index of < 0.90, i.e. systolic blood pressure of the arm intended for vascular access creation divided by the systolic blood pressure of the contralateral arm) is indicative of proximal arterial obstructive disease. In these cases, surgical or radiological intervention for the underlying cause should be performed before creating an A/V fistula.
- Examination of peripheral arteries
  The pulse of the brachial artery is palpated at the medial side of the elbow, the radial and ulnar arteries are palpated 2 cm proximal of the processus styloideus radii and proc. styloideus ulnae, respectively. Calcified arteries are generally hard and non-pulsatile. A weak or absent pulse might indicate obstruction of the artery. Auscultation of the subclavian or axillary artery may reveal a bruit suggesting stenosis.
- The Allen-Test
  The patency of the distal radial and ulnar artery and the palmar arch can be examined by the Allen test[1, 2]. The radial and ulnar arterial refilling of the hand is examined by the selective compression and decompression of the radial and ulnar artery at the wrist. In the modified version, the patient is asked to clench the

fist, meanwhile both arteries are compressed. Then the fist is unclenched followed by release of the radial artery. Adequate hand perfusion results in a return of capillary refilling within 5 seconds. The test is then repeated but this time releasing the ulnar artery whilst keeping the radial artery compressed. In 1976, Kamienski et al. pointed out that to obtain results correlating with Doppler ultrasound measurements, the proper performance of the Allen test is essential, i.e. that there is no hyperextension of the wrist or the fingers as this may reduce bloodflow[3].

However, the accuracy of the Allen test to detect distal radial or ulnar artery occlusion is doubtful. Jarvis et al. correlated clinical examinations by means of the Allen test with Doppler examination of the radial and ulnar artery. With cut-off values of 3, 5 and 6 seconds for capillary refilling-time the sensitivity was 100 %, 76 % and 54 %, respectively, with a specificity of 27 %, 82 % and 92 %. The diagnostic accuracy was 52 %, 80 % and 79 %, respectively[4]

McGregor performed intra-arterial fluorescence angiography and found no correlation with clinical testing[5]. Inter-observer variation concerning the Allen test is also reported[6].

On the other hand some investigators found a good correlation between objective measurements (Doppler ultrasound or angiography) and clinical assessment of the distal wrist arteries, and considered it as useful in the diagnosis of the patency of the palmar arch, despite the high percentage of false negative results (almost 20 %)[7]. Others recommend it only as a primary screening method[8], whose accuracy can be increased by the use of laser-Doppler measurement, but not by pulse oximetry[9].

In conclusion, the Allen test is a subjective assessment of distal hand circulation with variable outcome. Therefore, it is not recommended in the assessment for AV fistula placement. Digital blood pressure monitoring has been described as an alternative to the Allen test[10].

1.2. Technical Methods

1.2.1. Iodine Venography

Iodine contrast media can cause a deterioration in renal function. Despite its possible nephrotoxicity, highly diluted iodine contrast material is still recommended by several authors for angiography and fistulography, as the amount needed (less than 5 ml) has virtually no effect on renal function. Digital subtraction angiography is preferred[11, 12].

1.2.2. CO_2 -Venography

In patients with severe iodine allergy or with poor renal function, CO_2-Venography may be an alternative. With CO_2 neither nephrotocixity nor allergic reactions are known. However the contrast between CO_2 and blood is lower than between iodine and blood. Thus, CO_2-Venography requires digital subtraction angiography.

The main risk in the use of CO_2-Venography is:
- Trapping of CO_2 in the right ventricle
- Trapping of CO_2 in the right ventricle may cause block (vapour lock) of the pulmonary outflow tract, thus leading to coronary ischaemia, bradycardia,

hypotension and possible death. To avoid this complication, the injected volume of CO_2 should be restricted to 50-100 ml per single injection (100 ml CO_2 at 4 bar is equivalent to 400 ml CO_2 at 1 bar pressure, Boyle's Law). Between each injection, 1 – 2 minutes should elapse to allow for CO_2 clearing by the lung.
If trapping of CO2 in the right ventricle has occurred, the right side of the patient should be elevated in order to lower the pulmonary artery and to move the CO_2 into the right atrium[12].

1.2.3. Gadolinum-Venography
Gadopentetate dimeglumine, a gadolinum-based contrast medium, adequately visualises the renal artery as well as veins of the upper extremity and central veins, if used with digital subtraction. It has been used safely in patients with severe pre-existing renal impairment and is thought to be less nephrotoxic than iodine contrast medium[13, 14] although this remains controversial[16].

1.2.4. Magnetic Resonance Angiography (MRA)
Peripheral and central veins have been successfully visualised by MRA, a non-invasive technique, which can also be performed with or without contrast media (Gadolinum) using the time-of-flight (TOF) technique. In the latter, veins with a diameter > 2 mm could be visualised[16]. MRA has been proven to be accurate and even superior to contrast venography for thoracic vessels[17].

1.2.5. Doppler Ultrasound
The Doppler ultrasound technique uses the Doppler effect - meaning that the frequency of sound waves change if they are reflected by a moving object. The change is dependent on the velocity of the object. Circulating blood cells (predominantly erythrocytes) reflect the ultrasound. Ultrasound can either be transformed into a sound that can be heard or visualised in a waveform.
Access flow can be measured by Doppler ultrasound with the caveat that Doppler techniques require laminar flow for accurate measurements of velocity whilst blood flow in a fistula is usually turbulent. Measurement must be performed at least 5 cm away from the A/V fistula anastomosis.

1.2.6. Duplex Colour-Coded Ultrasound
Duplex ultrasound is a combination of B-mode ultrasound, producing a two-dimensional picture of the anatomy, and of Doppler ultrasound. The velocity of the blood is shown using different colours for different velocities and different directions of blood flow. Blood flow in the vessel can also be calculated. Thus it is possible to visualise in a single screen both the anatomy and the blood flow in vessels.
Duplex Doppler flow measurements can be predictive of thrombosis, but the disadvantages are the great inter-observer and inter-device variability, the adequacy being dependent on the anatomic location of the access, and the high costs[18]. Colour coded duplex ultrasonography is able to replace angiography except for hand arteries and central veins[19].
Normal Doppler waveform (measured by pulse wave Doppler) of a peripheral artery shows "high resistance", with positive systolic velocity and negative

diastolic velocity. The feeding artery of an A/V fistula on the other hand shows a flow of "low resistance", with positive systolic (SV) and positive diastolic (DV) velocity. The resistance index (RI) can be calculated by:

RI = (SV-DV)/SV

Resistance index of a peripheral artery is normally above 1 and in a feeding A/V fistula artery < 1. At reactive hyperaemia, provoked by clenched fist for two minutes, "high resistance" flow of a peripheral artery (of the upper limb) is changed to "low resistance", and RI changes from >1 to < 1. This could be used as a test for functional characteristics of the artery, which should be used for the creation of an A/V fistula[20].

2. Vascular Access Creation

First choice are direct wrist A/V fistulas, second choice are autogenous A/V fistulas at the elbow - brachiocephalic, transposed brachiobasilic, and autogenous vein transfers[21].

2.1. Upper Limb – Forearm A/V Fistula

The most peripheral location of the A/V anastomosis provides an optimal length of vein for cannulation.

2.1.1. Radiocephalic Fistula

Brescia et al. in 1966 originally described a side-to-side radial artery-to-cephalic vein A/V fistula. Today, the end-of-vein to side-of-artery anastomosis is preferred, as the patency rate is similar but there is a lower incidence of venous hypertension of the hand compared to side-to-side fistulas[22]. The anastomosis is performed close to the wrist joint, if adequate vessels exist at this site.

Vein transposition, such as the forearm basilic or the long saphenous vein, increases the possibility of creating a forearm A/V fistula, however, the transposition of the vein can reduce its capacity to dilate and mature.

2.1.2. Other Forearm Fistulas

Less common are snuff-box radiocephalic fistulas (created in the anatomical snuff box between the tendons of extensor pollicis longus and extensor pollicis brevis)[23] and ulnar basilic fistula (created between the basilic vein and the ulnar artery at the wrist)[24].

2.2. Elbow/Antecubital Fistulas and Upper Arm A/V Fistula

If the creation of a forearm A/V fistula is deemed impossible, upper limb fistulas created at the elbow are the second choice. Controlled, randomised trials comparing upper arm A/V fistulas and prosthetic grafts are absent. Oliver et al. retrospectively analysed transposed brachiobasilic fistulas, upper arm grafts and brachiocephalic fistulas. They found higher thrombosis rates (50 % vs. 23 % at one year), higher infection rates (13 % to 0 %) and increased requirement for intervention (2.4 vs. 0.7 per access-year) in upper arm grafts compared to transposed brachiobasilic fistulas[25]. Therefore, creation of an upper-arm A/V fistula should be preferred to graft placement.

2.2.1. Brachiocephalic Fistula

Depending on the anatomy of the antecubital fossa several techniques are described to connect the brachial artery to the cephalic vein. The preferred method is the end-of-vein to side-of-artery configuration which reduces the risk of retrograde venous hypertension. This form of fistula may not be suitable for obese patients. Although technically possible, the vein may be located too deep to be needled easily in obese patients and the length of the arterialised vein may be too short. Resection of the fatty tissue can make needling easier. Reported patency rates are comparable to those observed in radiocephalic fistulas and range between 70 – 75 % after one year[26] to 80 % after 4.5 years[27]. The main complications are vein stenosis due to intimal hyperplasia, venous aneurysmal dilatation and vascular steal syndrome[26, 28, 29].

A special variant of elbow fistulae, the perforating vein fistula (PVF), was first described in 1977[30]. In many patients, the perforating vein seems to be the continuation of the cephalic vein. In contrast to the original technical procedure with partial resection of the deep venous system, it is nowadays preferred to preserve the continuity of the deep veins. The perforating vein is transected before entering the deep veins. That means, that the length of the A/V anastomosis is limited to the diameter of the perforating vein, typically 3 to 5 mm. This procedure can advantageously be used for creation of an elbow vascular access in diabetic, female and elderly patients[31]. A good arterialised cephalic vein provides for long-term cannulation due to its subcutaneous position.

A further possibility is the creation of a brachiocephalic bridge graft fistula. A PTFE graft (usually 6 mm in diameter) is anastomosed to the brachial artery and the cephalic vein[32].

2.2.2. Brachiobasilic Fistula with Transposed Vein

The anastomosis is constructed – if possible – at the level of the elbow using the median basilic vein, generally as an end-of vein to side-of-artery anastomosis. Special attention should be paid to the length of the anastomosis which should not exceed the diameter of the brachial artery by more than 2 mm and should never be more than 7 mm in total, otherwise the risk of steal syndrome will increase substantially. Recent publications recommend a subcutaneous superficialisation of the basilic vein up to the level of the axilla[25]. However, it might be advantageous to transpose only a segment leading to a cannulation area of 8 - 10 cm, in order to preserve the cephalad segment of the non-transposed basilic vein for future procedures.

If this technique is used without prior arterialisation of the vein, there may be a higher failure rate. A two-step procedure is recommended by performing the initial anastomosis and then transposing the basilic vein after an interval of 4-8 weeks, in order to allow sufficient time for maturation and blood flow rates of the 500 or 600 ml/min may be measured by ultrasound. In a patient with a pre-dilated basilic vein, transposition can be performed as a one stage procedure.

Brachiobasilic fistulas can also be performed at the level of the elbow in a side-of-vein to side-of-artery fashion. Thus, all the veins at the elbow, proximal and distal to the anastomosis are available for dialysis. In order to avoid venous hypertension and steal syndrome, the arterial anastomosis should not be more than 7 mm in length[33].

2.3. Lower Limb Vascular Access

If all vessels in the upper limb are no longer suitable for vascular access creation, a vascular access in the lower limb serves as alternative. Multiple surgical approaches have been used to create a lower limb vascular access. We recommend saphenous vein and superficial femoral vein transposition and superficialisation. Contra-indication for lower limb access are advanced peripheral arterial disease or critical ischaemia, including critical ischaemia stage III/IV (Leriche-Fontaine classification). Atherosclerosis will be indicated by the absence of distal pulses in the foot and popliteal fossa. In these cases, the ankle-brachial pressure index should be determined. An index < 0.9 suggests peripheral vascular disease with the possibility of an elevated risk of limb ischaemia and steal-syndrome after creation of a vascular access.

Due to the greater diameter of the vessels, patency rates are in general better than in upper limb A/V fistula. On the other hand, the high flow rates, especially in combination with atherosclerosis of the vessels, carry the risk of steal syndrome and ischaemia. In addition, leg oedema might occur in case of venous obstruction. Some authors find higher rates of infection in vascular accesses in the lower limb compared to those in the upper limb, whilst others have not[34].

2.4. Grafts for Vascular Access

Primary use of prosthetic material for vascular access is not recommended because of its high frequency of complications. Such material should only be used if there is no possibility of the creation of a autogenous A/V-fistula. Vascular access can be created using bio-grafts and synthetic grafts, to connect an adequate artery with an adequate vein.

Bio-grafts can be divided into:
Autografts: Generally the long saphenous vein or superficial femoral vein of the patient is used and either transplanted to the arm or transposed in the leg.
Allografts: Cryopreserved saphenous or femoral veins may become the graft material of the future. Veins obtained from patients after varicose vein stripping are rarely used nowadays because of the risk of HIV infection although they have been used in the past.
Xenografts: Today, bovine mesenteric veins (Procol®) and sheep ovine veins (Omniflow®) are used as xenograft. They are denaturated and in case of synthetic grafts are made from several different materials:
PTFE: Polytetrafluoroethylene is made from Teflon. The expanded PTFE (ePTFE) is composed of solid nodes, connected by thin fibres.
Dacron: Dacron may be a woven or knitted porous graft made from polyester.
Leakage through the graft can be prevented by pre-clotting or coating with collagen or gelatin.
Polyurethane graft: Polyurethane has a spongy structure that is microporous. Due to its compliance, it may inhibit intimal hyperplasia, thereby reducing stenosis rates.

2.5. Catheters and Ports

Catheters used for dialysis can be divided into:
1. Tunneled or non-tunneled catheters
2. Single or dual-lumen catheters
3. Polyurethane or silicone catheters

Catheters for dialysis may be used in cases of acute renal failure or when the catheter will be restricted to 2-3 weeks. Single and dual-lumen catheters can be used. Catheters which are relatively stiff have been associated with perforation of vessels and of the right atrium and should be avoided[35].

In dual-lumen catheters, the lines ought not be reversed, as this increases the recirculation of blood, thus reducing the efficiency of dialysis, although sometimes this is unavoidable[36]. Level et al. described an increase in recirculation from 2.9 +/- 5 to 12 +/- 9 % in reversing the blood lines[37].
Catheters can also be made from different materials. While silicone is incompatible with tincture of iodine and may be degraded by povidone-iodine, polyurethane catheters are incompatible with alcohols including isopropyl alcohol, and ointments containing polyethylene glycol (PEG)[38].

Currently there is insufficient data to recommend the use of ports as opposed to catheters. Ports[39] or similar systems like Dialock®[40] and LifeSite®[41] are alternatives to permanent tunneled catheters. These totally subcutaneous vascular access devices may reduce the rate of infection, since the skin barrier remains intact. They offer higher blood flow rates than catheters[41]. A high acceptance by the patients has been reported, as they are less visible and allow bathing. However, the devices and the special cannulae needed for puncture are costly.

Appendix

3. Monitoring

Early detection of stenosis of the vascular access and intervention increases patency rates of the vascular access[18, 42, 43, 44]. A correct technique for the measurement of recirculation, static or dynamic venous pressure is essential to achieve reliable results:

3.1. Urea Based Measurement of Recirculation (Slow-Flow-Technique)
Procedure[45]
- Measure during the first 30 min of dialysis
- Turn off ultrafiltration
- Draw blood samples for urea determination from the arterial and venous blood lines
    - A = concentration of urea in the arterial line with possible recirculation
    - V = concentration of urea in the venous line after the blood has been dialysed
- Reduce blood pump to 50 ml/min
- Exactly 15 to 25 seconds later draw another blood sample S from the arterial line port
    - S = concentration of urea in the arterial line without recirculation
- Resume dialysis
- Recirculation in % = (S – A) / (S – V) x 100
    - with S – A = reduction in the urea concentration caused by recirculation
    - S – V = reduction in the urea concentration caused by dialysis

3.2. Static Intra-Access Venous Pressure (SVP)
Procedure[46]
- Measure mean arterial blood pressure (MAP) in the contralateral arm
- Open venous clamp manually and stop blood pump for 30 seconds
- Determine the arterial and venous offset pressure (Po_{ffa} and Po_{ffv}) between access site and pressure sensor:
    - Measure the height difference A in cm between access and fluid level in the arterial pressure line. Po_{ffa} in mm Hg = A x 0.75
    - Measure the height difference V in cm between access and fluid level in the venous drip chamber. Po_{ffv} in mm Hg = V x 0.75
    (leading to a Po_{ff} > 0 mm Hg, if access arm is below fluid level (normal case), or to a Po_{ff} < 0 mm Hg, if access arm is above fluid level (height is then negative)
- Read the venous and arterial pressure (PA, PV) after pressure relaxation in the pressure display of your dialysis machine
- Calculate the static arterial and venous intra-access pressure ratio SPR_a and SPR_v:
    SPR_a = (PA + Po_{ffa})/MAP
    SPR_v = (PV + Po_{ffv})/MAP

3.3. Dynamic Venous Pressure (DVP)
Procedure:
- Use 15 gauge needle size
- During the first 5 min of each dialysis session raise the blood flow to 200 ml/min.

At higher flow rates, there is excessive turbulence at the level of the dialysis needle and the pressure readings loses its predictive capacity.
– Read DVP from the venous pressure display in your machine
– Proposed threshold to order angiography is dependent on the machine. Pressures regarded as elevated are:
  – a DVP > 100 - 150 mm Hg in 3 consecutive readings[42, 43] **or**
  – a DVP > 125 mm Hg with a blood flow of 200 ml/min[45] resp. a DVP > 150 mm Hg in standard blood flow for the patient[43]
– Pressures must be consistently elevated in three consecutive dialysis to avoid errors caused by needle placement.

3.4. Vascular Access Blood Flow Measurement with Reversed Lines

3.4.1. Ultrasound dilution
– Puncture the fistula with the arterial cannula against the flow direction of the vascular access
– An injection port must be integrated in the venous blood line
– Clip arterial line flow/dilution sensor onto arterial blood line and venous sensor onto the venous line
– Reverse the lines for access flow measurement by cross connecting the venous blood line to the arterial needle tubing and vice versa
– Choose an effective blood flow Q_b between 200 and 300 ml/min
– Extend the limits of the venous pressure to avoid pump stoppage during infusion
– Draw 10 ml of physiologic saline into a sterile syringe and inject it within 3 to 5 seconds into the venous blood line
– Determine recirculation RX from dilution data (e.g. a RX of 25 % is equal to 0.25)
– Calculate access blood flow Q_a:

$$Q_a = Q_b \cdot \left(\frac{1}{RX} - 1 \right)$$

3.4.2. Thermodilution
– Puncture the fistula with the arterial cannula against the flow direction of the vascular access
– Choose an effective blood flow Q_b of at least 200 ml/min and stop ultrafiltration
– Measure recirculation RN in normal blood line position (e.g. a value of 5 % is equal to 0.05)
– Stop blood flow and reverse the lines for access flow measurement by cross connecting the venous blood line to the arterial needle tubing and vice versa
– Restore effective blood flow Q_b and measure recirculation RX with reversed blood lines
– Calculate access blood flow Q_a:

3.5. Check-box for assessment of vascular access at each dialysis session:

$$Qa = Qb \cdot \left(\frac{1 - RX - RN + RX * RN}{RX - RN} \right)$$

The check-box below is an example and should be adopted to local requirements and to the vascular access used in the respective patient.

	Finding	Date	Action	Result / Outcome
	Monitoring at each dialysis session			
✓	**Physical examination**			
✓	Abnormal bruit or thrill			
✓	Signs of infection			
✓	Swollen limb			
✓	Aneurysm / pseudoaneurysm			
✓	Ischaemia stage 3 (rest pain) or 4 (necrosis)			
✓	**Cannulation problems**			
✓	Difficult cannulation			
✓	Aspirating clot			
✓	Prolonged bleeding			
✓	**Problems during HD**			
✓	Increased dynamic venous pressure			
✓	Arterial line pressure < - 250 mm Hg			
✓	Inability to supply prescribed Q_b			
	Monitoring monthly			
✓	Decreased access flow			
✓	Increased static venous pressure			
✓	Recirculation			

4. Treatment of Stenosis and Thrombosis

4.1. Interventional Options

4.1.1. PTA

4.1.1.1. Dilatation technique[47]

Regular dilatation is an outpatient procedure. An antegrade venous approach should be used for stenoses located far enough from the arterial anastomosis, and a retrograde approach should be used for stenoses close to the arterial anastomosis. An 18G needle and a 0.035 inch guide wire offer good support for placement of a 6 to 9 F introducer sheath. A short subcutaneous tunnel between the skin entry-point and the fistula or graft entry-point will facilitate the final compression and decrease the risk of pseudo-aneurysm formation.

Once a guide wire has passed through the stenosis, heparin may be injected (2,000 to 3,000 units) but it is necessary only in small diameter or low flow fistulae.

Usually the diameter of the dilatation balloon should be equal to or 1 mm greater than the diameter of the immediately upstream or downstream normal vessel (choose 1 mm above the smaller one in cases of discrepancy).

The balloon is inflated with a manometer filled with contrast medium diluted to 75 %. Pressure is slowly increased to abolish the waist of the stenosis on the balloon, the edges of which must be completely parallel. The inflated balloon is left in place for 1 to 3 minutes. Dilatation is often painful locally. Local anaesthesia can be performed when stenoses are just under the skin. Neurolept analgesia may otherwise be necessary.

Haemodialysis access stenoses are often very hard and high pressure balloons with bursting pressures of over 25 atmospheres are often necessary. Immediate post-dilatation angiography, with the guide wire left in place through the dilated area, may show several possibilities:

- No residual stenosis and no wall damage: The procedure is then completed.
- Minor vein wall damage: 3 to 5 minutes low pressure ballooning is performed to try to smooth out the vessel wall.
- Rupture with clear extravasation of contrast medium and haematoma: The balloon must be re-inflated rapidly to 2 atmospheres for repeated periods of 10 minutes.
- Residual stenosis: If there is no vein wall damage, a new dilatation is performed with a longer inflation time (3 min) with a balloon which is 1 mm greater in diameter. At this stage, a less than 30 % residual stenosis is acceptable only if it results from the first dilatation ever performed in this stenosis. If there is greater than 30 % residual stenosis, a new dilatation should be performed with a larger balloon but more than 2 mm over-dilatation is not recommended. Stenosis recoil is possible, especially in central veins, and should be treated by stent placement.

Once the dilatation has been performed, the catheters and introducer sheath are removed. The puncture site must be compressed as gently as possible to stop bleeding without stopping flow through the fistula. The procedure is thus completed and the vascular access is immediately usable for haemodialysis.

4.1.1.2. Specific cases[47]
- Stenoses resistant to 25 bar pressures are infrequent. Atherectomy catheters [6], cutting balloons[7] or the Redha-cut (Sheringmed, Switzerland) have been reported to be of some value in such cases.
- Arm oedema is due to stenosis or occlusion of a central vein (subclavian or brachio-cephalic) and is the consequence of previous central catheters. In chronic occlusion, it may be necessary to use a double approach via the femoral vein and via the fistula in order to traverse the occluded lumen successfully.
- Stenoses of the feeding artery and of the arterio-venous anastomosis may be impossible to traverse using a regular retrograde fistula approach. Antegrade puncture of the brachial artery and catheterisation of the feeding artery is feasible.

4.1.1.3. Contra-indications to dilatation[47]
- Absolute contra-indications
  Local infection
  Concomitant arterial steal syndrome
- Relative contra-indications
  Surgical anastomoses of less than 6 weeks are at high risk of rupture. Gentle dilatation at low pressure with an exact size-matched diameter balloon can however be contemplated at venous anastomoses of grafts.
  Immature (< 2 months) fistulas are indications for surgery if the stenosis is located in the anastomotic area. However, when the underlying stenosis is located far from the anastomosis, gentle dilatation is the simplest method to save the fistula.
  Isolated stenosis within 5 cm of the wrist in a Brescia-Cimino fistula can be dilated but should preferably be treated surgically.
  Long (> 5 cm) stenoses and chronic occlusions at the venous anastomoses of grafts and in upper arm cephalic veins usually provide poor results and surgical revision should be undertaken.
  High flow is mainly a complication of upper arm fistulae and is a contra-indication for dilatation because the treatment of the stenosis would increase the already high flow.

4.1.1.4. Stents[48]
Indications for stent placement must be restricted, and only self-expandable stents should be placed in dialysis access. Covered stents are only recommended for rupture control. Stent diameter must be at least 1 to 2 mm greater than the diameter of the largest balloon used for dilatation, its length should be as short as possible. Stent patency is limited because stenosis recurs either within the stent or at its ends. In order not to interfere with future access creation, stent placement is contraindicated at the venous anastomosis of a forearm graft if the stent would overlap the basilic vein. Equally, a stent placed in the final arch of the cephalic vein should not protrude into the subclavian vein, a stent placed in the subclavian vein must not overlap the ostium of a patent internal jugular vein, and finally a stent placed in the right of left brachio-cephalic ("innominate") vein must not protrude into the superior vena cava.

4.1.2. Percutaneous Declotting[49]

Percutaneous declotting of thrombosed autogenous and prosthetic arterio-venous access can be accomplished by a variety of pharmacological, pharmaco-mechanical, and mechanical approaches.

4.1.2.1. Pharmacological Thrombolysis

Pharmacological declotting basically means injection of a thrombolytic agent into the thrombosed access. The procedure should always be combined with treatment of the underlying stenosis, since complete lysis and patency rates following thrombolysis only have been disappointing.

4.1.2.2. Pharmaco-mechanical Thrombolysis

Pharmaco-mechanical thrombolysis is composed of two phases. First pharmacological lysis of the thrombus takes place followed immediately by mechanical maceration and removal of residual thrombus and by dilatation of residual stenosis. When combined with consequent treatment of all stenoses, immediate success rates of more than 90 % can be achieved.

4.1.2.3. Mechanical Declotting

Purely mechanical methods include the balloon-based methods of Trerotola and Sharaffuddin, manual catheter-directed thromboaspiration, the saline pulse-spray technique of Beathard, the Gelbfish device, the rotating pigtail of Schmitz-Rode and several types of declotting machines. Among these machines, some have a direct action (Arrow-Trerotola PTD®, Cragg brush®) but the majority work on the Venturi effect or on the creation of a vortex (Hydrolyser®, Amplatz-Thrombectomy Device®, Angiojet®, Oasis®), and many others are likely to be marketed . No method or device can claim to work better than another but there are difference in costs and in the size of particles pushed into the lungs[48].

4.2. Surgical Options

All surgical corrective procedures can be performed in an outpatient setting and under local or regional anaesthesia. Before clamping the access, 3,000 to 5,000 IU heparin are administered. At the end of the operation, after de-clotting the access, protamine can be given to reverse heparin effect (beware of the possibility of hypotension after protamine administration in insulin-dependent diabetics).

4.2.1. Proximal Re-anastomosis

Fistula vein stenosis is very often found close to the arterio-venous anastomosis in forearm fistulas. After ligation of the vein in its stenosed segment, a new side-to-end anastomosis immediately proximal to the stenosis can be performed using standard techniques as for primary access construction. In most cases, this secondary procedure is much easier than the primary one, because after some months or years of fistula function, artery and vein will be significantly dilated. Although published experience is limited, proximal re-anastomosis is believed to provide better patency rates than PTA[47].

4.2.2. Patch Angioplasty

Less frequently, stenoses of the needling segment of the fistula vein will compromise fistula function. In the case of a stenosed wrist access very proximal re-anastomosis can result in significant loss of access length. Therefore, in short stenoses, surgical patch angioplasty will be the better alternative[9], because the complete access is preserved. Patch angioplasty can also be performed in anastomotic stenoses of prosthetic access.

The vein or graft-to-vein anastomosis is exposed through a longitudinal skin incision and opened longitudinally after clamping proximal and distal to the stenosis. The incision must begin and end in a vein (graft) segment with "normal" calibre. A segment of the long saphenous vein or a synthetic patch are used for closure of the venotomy or graft incision.

4.2.3. Graft Interposition

In stenoses of the needling segment of autogenous or prosthetic access longer than 4 or 5 cm, interposition grafting is easier and quicker than suturing a long patch[50, 51]. The access is exposed through two separate incisions proximally and distally to the stenosis. After clamping, the vessel or graft is transected leaving the stenosed segment in place. In autogenous access the long saphenous vein may serve as interposition graft provided it is of adequate diameter and length. In fistula veins dilated to 6 mm or more and in grafts, graft interposition will probably give more satisfactory results. The graft is positioned in a subcutaneous tunnel past the stenotic needling site and sutured end-to-end to both the proximal and distal end of the transected vein or graft.

4.2.4. Graft Extension

Stenoses of the venous anastomosis of prosthetic access longer than 4 or 5 cm or complete occlusions of the post-anastomotic vein is bridged by graft extension. The graft is exposed close to its venous anastomosis as is the draining vein upward of the occlusion. After clamping and transecting the graft, an end-to-end anastomosis is sutured with the extension graft, which is then tunneled into the incision over the vein. When the new graft has to bridge a joint region to reach the draining vein, great care must be taken to find a position where it is not kinked during joint movement or a ringed graft used[52]. The anastomosis to the vein is sutured in an end-to-side fashion after a longitudinal venotomy.

4.2.5. Surgical Thrombectomy

Simultaneous correction of the underlying access stenosis is an integral part of surgical thrombectomy. Therefore the thrombosed vein or graft is exposed through a skin incision at a location allowing for adequate access to the presumed site of the stenosis. This means that if open surgical correction is planned, the incision is made over or close to the suspected area of stenosis. When an endovascular procedure is performed, the incision is made at reasonable distance from the presumed stenosis to allow for easy handling of the introducer sheath and all necessary interventional equipment. The vein or graft is opened transversely, and the thrombus is extracted with an embolectomy catheter of adequate diameter. In tortuous or aneurysmal veins, remaining thrombus can be mobilised and even be expressed by digital massage. Treatment of stenoses is performed with standard surgical or endovascular techniques as described above. Completion on-table angiography is mandatory regardless of whether open surgical or endovascular correction of the access stenosis was performed.

5. Vascular Access Infections in Dialysis Patients

Infection causes 15 to 36 % of all-cause mortality in haemodialysis patients, a 100 to 300 fold higher risk of death caused by sepsis in ESRD patients when compared to the general population[53, 54].

Vascular access infections are implicated as the cause of 48 % to 73 % of all bacteraemia in haemodialysis patients[53]. The majority of bacteraemia is caused by staphylococcal organisms[53, 55]. Bacteraemia is associated with high rates of mortality (8 to 25 %) and recurrence (14 to 44 %) and metastatic complications (14 to 44 %, average 25 %[53], amongst which are infectious endocarditis, septic arthritis, epidural abscess, septic pulmonary emboli and osteomyelitis. The risk is higher with S. aureus infection[56].

5.1. Infections in Different Types of Vascular Accesses

5.1.1. Infections Related to Tunneled (Cuffed) Catheters

Bacteraemia is much more frequent in patients with central venous catheters than in patients with A/V fistula, with a relative risk (RR) of 7.6[57]. Infection-related deaths are also more frequent in patients with central venous catheters, with a 2.3 RR in patients with diabetes mellitus and 1.83 RR in patients without diabetes mellitus, compared to patients with A/V fistula[58].

In 1988, Schwab et al. inserted eighty tunneled cuffed catheters. They reported only one case of bacteraemia in 4480 catheter-days, corresponding to 0.22 per 1000 catheter-days[59]. However, randomised studies comparing cuffed and noncuffed catheters are rare. A non-randomised study was performed by Jean et al., who followed up 62 double-cuffed catheters without lateral holes and 63 non-cuffed catheters with lateral holes, both inserted with creation of a tunnel. Bacteraemia occurred in 1.3 per 1000 catheter-days in cuffed and 1.08 per 1000 catheter-days in non-cuffed catheters. Similar, local infection rates were higher in cuffed than in non-cuffed catheters (1.3 to 0.77 per 1000 catheter-days respectively)[60]. Similarly, higher risk for access related bacteraemia per 1000 catheter-days was reported by the Center for Disease Control (Atlanta, USA) for cuffed (2.91) than for non-cuffed catheters (1.6)[61].

In tunneled cuffed catheters Beathard et al., Marr et al. and Saad reported 3.4, 3.8 and 5.5 catheter related bacteraemia per 1000 catheter-days, respectively[56, 62, 63]. These higher rates compared to those mentioned above may be explained by different catheter handling procedures. Beathard et al. described a decrease in catheter-related bacteraemia from 4.7 to 1.6 per 1000 catheter-days after changes in the protocol for catheter management[62].

Among temporary catheters, femoral catheters are more susceptible to infections than those in thoracic location, and internal jugular have higher infection rates than subclavian[64, 65]. However, these results do not justify use of the subclavian vein catheterisation, since subclavian vein catheters carry the highest risk of central vein stenosis[66].

Colonisation of catheters occurs most frequently through the lumen at the time of connecting the hub to dialysis blood lines, and not by migration of bacteria down the outer surface of the catheter[67].

The presence of a biofilm on the inner and outer surface of the catheter may play an important role in catheter-related bacteraemia. Bacteria adhere and become embedded in the glycocalyx of the biofilm making them more resistant to antibiotics than those floating in the circulation[68].

Frequent destruction of the endoluminal biofilm by means of a fibrinolytic agent and local instillation of antibiotics left in situ (antiseptic lock) may be an effective means for the prevention of a blood stream infection.

5.1.2. Infections of the PTFE Graft and the A/V Fistula

PTFE grafts have a high risk of infection beginning at surgical placement, with a 6 % initial 30 days infection rate or even higher in the femoral location. The risk of infection in grafts is much higher than in A/V fistulas[69, 70]. Likewise, the relative risk of infection-related deaths is 2.47 for patients with diabetes, and 1.27 for patients without diabetes, compared to patients with an A/V fistula[58].

5.2. Antibiotic Treatment

Empirical antibiotic treatment must cover both gram positive, responsible for up to 75 % of catheter-related infections, and gram negative organisms. Resistance to antibiotics is also a problem in catheter-related bacteraemia in dialysis patients. About 40 – 75 % of gram positive bacteraemia is methicillin resistant. Some species of S. aureus are not only resistant to methicillin but also show a decreased susceptibility to glycopeptides[71].

Aiming to cover both gram positive and negative organisms in empirical treatment for suspected infection of haemodialysis vascular access, and, considering the high incidence of MRSA, and the convenient pharmacokinetics of vancomycin in ESRD, it has become common practice to combine vancomycin 1g i.v. (or 20 mg/kg) every 5 to 7 days plus gentamycin 80 mg (1 to 2 mg/kg) every 24 to 48 hours, thus allowing outpatient prolonged parenteral antibiotic treatment. The use of high flux or large surface area dialysers may require vancomycin to be dosed after each treatment to maintain effective blood levels. In this setting a dosing schedule of 500 mg of vancomycin after each dialysis session may be more appropriate[71].

The empirical use of this combination is still justified in severe infections with bacteraemia, fever or blood pressure instability.

With the emergence of vancomycin-resistant enterococci and the justifiable concern of induction of vancomycin resistant staphylococci, empirical use of vancomycin for the febrile patient on hemodialysis has recently been challenged by several authorities[72, 73]. The Center of Disease Control and Prevention (CDC) suggested vancomycin to be reserved for b-lactam allergy or for serious infection where ß-lactam resistant gram-positive bacteria (MRSA, Staphylococci epidermidis) are likely.

The European Best Practice Guidelines on Haemodialysis recommend the empirical use of methicillin, in order to avoid development of glycopeptide resistance.

They recommend vancomycin in settings with increased MRSA. In severely ill patients, a third or fourth generation cephalosporin should be added to cover gram-negative bacteria including Pseudomonas aeruginosa.

In dialysis units with a low rate of MRSA, or when antibiotic sensitivity is available, vancomycin can be safely and effectively substituted by cefazolin 20 mg/kg at the end of each dialysis treatment[74].

Most authorities, however, still recommend initial treatment with broad spectrum vancomycin plus aminoglycoside. Rapid conversion to cefazolin regimen or other appropriate antibiotics based on culture and sensitivities is needed, not only to prevent emergence of resistant organisms, but also to avoid ototoxicity.

Metastatic complications are more common with short courses of antimicrobial treatment (2 weeks or less). Therefore, in the case of bacteraemia, four weeks of adequate antibiotic treatment is advocated for S. aureus and a minimum of three weeks for all the other organisms[62, 75]. The EBPG recommend four weeks of antibiotics in all cases of bacteraemia.

Blood cultures should be repeated 1 week following the end of therapy to ensure that the infection has been eradicated[62].

References see p. 156

References

Most quoted papers have been graded according to the following three levels of evidence:

- Evidence level A: Meta-analysis of several randomised controlled trials
  Randomised controlled trials
- Evidence level B: Controlled study without randomisation
  Experimental study
  Comparative study
  Correlation study
  Case study
- Evidence level C: Expert report
  Opinion or clinical experience of respected authorities.

References – Starting Management of Vascular Access

1. Bonucchi D, Cappelli G, Albertazzi A. Which is the preferred vascular access in diabetic patients? A view from Europe. *Nephrol Dial Transplant* 2002; 17:20-22 (evidence level: C)
2. Konner K. Venous Preservation. *Blood Purif* 2002; 19:115 (evidence level: C)
3. Schwab SJ, Quarles LD, Middleton JP, Cohan RH, Saeed M, Dennis VW. Hemodialysis-associated subclavian vein stenosis. *Kidney Int* 1988; 33:1156-1159 (evidence level: B)
4. Van Biesen W, Vanholder RC, Veys N, Dhondt A, Lameire NH. An evaluation of an integrative care approach for end-stage renal disease patients. *J Am Soc Nephrol* 2000; 11:116-125 (evidence level: B)
5. Jungers P, Massy ZA, Nguyen-Khoa T, Choukroun G, Robino C, Fakhouri F, Touam M, Nguyen AT, Grunfeld JP. Longer duration of predialysis nephrological care is associated with improved long-term survival of dialysis patients. *Nephrol Dial Transplant* 2001; 16:2357-2364 (evidence level: B)
6. Besarab A, Adams M, Amatucci S, Bowe D, Deane J, Ketchen K, Reynolds K, Tello A. Unraveling the realities of vascular access: the Network 11 experience. *Adv Ren Replace Ther* 2000; 7:S65-S70 (evidence level: B)
7. Beckingham IJ, O'Rourke JS, Bishop MC, Blamey RW. Are backup arteriovenous fistulae necessary for patients on continuous ambulatory peritoneal dialysis? *Lancet* 1993; 341:1384-1386 (evidence level: B)
8. Mujais S, Nolph K, Gokal R, Blake P, Burkart J, Coles G, Kawaguchi Y, Kawanishi H, Korbet S, Krediet R, Lindholm B, Oreopoulos D, Rippe B, Selgas R. Evaluation and management of ultrafiltration problems in peritoneal dialysis. International Society for Peritoneal Dialysis Ad Hoc Committee on Ultrafiltration Management in Peritoneal Dialysis. *Perit Dial Int* 2000; 20 Suppl 4:S5-21 (evidence level: C)

References – Patient with Acute Need for Dialysis Access

1. Schwab SJ and Beathard G. The hemodialysis catheter conundrum: hate living with them, but can't live without them. *Kidney Int* 1999; 56:1-17 (evidence level: C)

2. Oliver MJ. Acute dialysis catheters. *Semin Dial* 2001; 14:432-435 (evidence level: C)
3. Kirkpatrick WG, Culpepper RM, Sirmon MD. Frequency of complications with prolonged femoral vein catheterization for hemodialysis access. *Nephron* 1996; 73: 58-62
4. Al Wakeel JS, Milwalli AH, Malik GH, Huraib S, Al-Mohaya S, Abu-Aisha H, Memon N. Dual-lumen femoral vein catheterization as vascular access for hemodialysis-a prospective study. *Angiology* 1998; 49: 557-562
5. Oliver MJ, Callery SM, Thorpe KE, Schwab SJ, Churchill DN. Risk of bacteremia from temporary hemodialysis catheters by site of insertion and duration of use: a prospective study. *Kidney Int* 2000; 58: 2543-2545
6. Kimata N, Nitta K, Akiba T, Tominaga K, Suzuki K, Watanabe Y, Haga T, Kawashima A, Miwa N, Nishida E, Aoki T, Nihei H.. Catheter dysfunction and thrombosis of double-lumen hemodialysis catheters placed in the femoral vein. *Clin Nephrol* 2002; 58: 215-219
7. Depner TA, Rizwan S, Stasi TA. Pressure effects on roller pump blood flow during hemodialysis. *ASAIO Trans* 1990; 36:M456-M459 (evidence level: B)
8. Trerotola SO, Johnson MS, Harris VJ, Shah H, Ambrosius WT, McKusky MA, Kraus MA. Outcome of tunneled hemodialysis catheters placed via the right internal jugular vein by interventional radiologists. *Radiology* 1997; 203:489-495 (evidence level: B)
9. Marr KA, Sexton DJ, Conlon PJ, Corey GR, Schwab SJ, Kirkland KB. Catheter-related bacteremia and outcome of attempted catheter salvage in patients undergoing hemodialysis. *Ann Intern Med* 1997; 127:275-280 (evidence level: B)
10. Saad TF. Bacteremia associated with tunneled, cuffed hemodialysis catheters. *Am J Kidney Dis* 1999; 34:1114-1124 (evidence level: B)

References – Clinical Evaluation of Access Site

1. Miller PE, Tolwani A, Luscy CP, Deierhoi MH, Bailey R, Redden DT, Allon M. Predictors of adequacy of arteriovenous fistulas in hemodialysis patients. *Kidney Int* 1999; 56:275-280 (evidence level: B)
2. Konner K. Increasing the proportion of diabetics with AV fistulas. *Semin Dial* 2001; 14:1-4 (evidence level: C)
3. Konner K. Primary vascular access in diabetic patients: an audit. *Nephrol Dial Transplant* 2000; 15:1317-1325 (evidence level: B)
4. Lazarides MK, Georgiadis GS, Tzilalis VD. Diabetes should not preclude efforts for creation of a primary radiocephalic fistula. *Nephrol Dial Transplant* 2002; 17:1852-1854
5. Sedlacek M, Teodorescu V, Falk A, Vassalotti JA, Uribarri J. Hemodialysis access placement with preoperative noninvasive vascular mapping: comparison between patients with and without diabetes. *Am J Kidney Dis* 2001; 38:560-564
6. Allon M, Lockhart ME, Lilly RZ, Gallichio MH, Young CJ, Barker J, Deierhoi MH, Robbin ML. Effect of preoperative sonographic mapping on vascular access outcomes in hemodialysis patients. *Kidney Int* 2001; 60:2013-2020 (evidence level: B)
7. Konner K and Vorwerk D. Permanent pacemaker wires causing subclavian vein stenosis in presence of AV fistula is it ever wrong to try angioplasty and stenting? *Nephrol Dial Transplant* 1997; 12:1735-1738 (evidence level: B)

8. Schillinger F, Schillinger D, Montagnac R, Milcent T. Post catheterisation vein stenosis in haemodialysis: comparative angiographic study of 50 subclavian and 50 internal jugular accesses. Nephrol Dial Transplant 1991; 6:722-724 (evidence level: B)
9. Konner K. When insufficient arterial inflow becomes the Achilles heel of the av-fistula - what are the surgical approaches? *Nephrol Dial Transplant* 2000; 15:145-147 (evidence level: C)
10. Malovrh M. Non-invasive evaluation of vessels by duplex sonography prior to construction of arteriovenous fistulas for haemodialysis. *Nephrol Dial Transplant* 1998; 13:125-129 (evidence level: B)
11. Sidawy AN, Gray R, Besarab A, Henry M, Ascher E, Silva M, Jr., Miller A, Scher L, Trerotola S, Gregory RT, Rutherford RB, Kent KC. Recommended standards for reports dealing with arteriovenous hemodialysis accesses. *J Vasc Surg* 2002; 35:603-610 (evidence level: C)
12. Silva MB, Jr., Hobson RW, Pappas PJ, Jamil Z, Araki CT, Goldberg MC, Gwertzman G, Padberg FT, Jr. A strategy for increasing use of autogenous hemodialysis access procedures: impact of preoperative noninvasive evaluation. *J Vasc Surg* 1998; 27:302-307 (evidence level: B)

References – Placement of Forearm A/V Fistula

1. Konner K. Primary vascular access in diabetic patients: an audit. *Nephrol Dial Transplant* 2000; 15:1317-1325 (evidence level: B)
2. Konner K. Increasing the proportion of diabetics with AV fistulas. *Semin Dial* 2001; 14:1-4 (evidence level: C)
3. Konner K, Hulbert-Shearon TE, Roys EC, Port FK. Tailoring the initial vascular access for dialysis patients. *Kidney Int* 2002; 62:329-338
4. Erasmi H, Horscch S., Schmidt R, Pichlmaier. Complications of arteriovenous fistulas and surgical intervention. *Lancester MTP Press Limited* 1984; 163-167 (evidence level: B)
5. Tordoir JH, Kwan TS, Herman JM, Carol EJ, Jakimowicz JJ. Primary and secondary access surgery for haemodialysis with the Brescia-Cimino fistula and the polytetrafluoroethylene (PTFE) graft. *Neth J Surg* 1983; 35:8-12 (evidence level: B)
6. Louridas G, Botha JR, Levien L, Milne FJ, Meyers AM, Myburgh JA. Vascular access for haemodialysis-experience at Johannesburg Hospital. *S Afr Med J* 1984; 66:637-640 (evidence level: B)
7. Wedgwood KR, Wiggins PA, Guillou PJ. A prospective study of end-to-side vs. side-to-side arteriovenous fistulas for haemodialysis. *Br J Surg* 1984; 71:640-642 (evidence level: A)
8. Palder SB, Kirkman RL, Whittemore AD, Hakim RM, Lazarus JM, Tilney NL. Vascular access for hemodialysis. Patency rates and results of revision. *Ann Surg* 1985; 202:235-239 (evidence level: B)
9. Kherlakian GM, Roedersheimer LR, Arbaugh JJ, Newmark KJ, King LR. Comparison of autogenous fistula versus expanded polytetrafluoroethylene graft fistula for angioaccess in hemodialysis. *Am J Surg* 1986; 152:238-243 (evidence level: B)
10. Mihmanli I, Besirli K, Kurugoglu S, Atakir K, Haider S, Ogut G, Numan F, Canturk E, Sayin AG. Cephalic vein and hemodialysis fistula: surgeon's observation versus color Doppler ultrasonographic findings. *J Ultrasound Med* 2001; 20:217-222 (evidence level: A)

11. Silva MB, Jr., Hobson RW, Pappas PJ, Jamil Z, Araki CT, Goldberg MC, Gwertzman G, Padberg FT, Jr. A strategy for increasing use of autogenous hemodialysis access procedures: impact of preoperative noninvasive evaluation. *J Vasc Surg* 1998; 27:302-307 (evidence level: B)
12. Malovrh M. Non-invasive evaluation of vessels by duplex sonography prior to construction of arteriovenous fistulas for haemodialysis. *Nephrol Dial Transplant* 1998; 13:125-129 (evidence level: B)
13. Robbin ML, Gallichio MH, Deierhoi MH, Young CJ, Weber TM, Allon M. US vascular mapping before hemodialysis access placement. *Radiology* 2000; 217:83-88 (evidence level: B)
14. Lemson MS, Leunissen KM, Tordoir JH. Does pre-operative duplex examination improve patency rates of Brescia-Cimino fistulas? *Nephrol Dial Transplant* 1998; 13:1360-1361 (evidence level: C)
15. Wladis AR, Mesh CL, White J, Zenni GC, Fischer DB, Arbaugh JJ. Improving longevity of prosthetic dialysis grafts in patients with disadvantaged venous outflow. *J Vasc Surg* 2000; 32:997-1005 (evidence level: B)
16. Yerdel MA, Kesenci M, Yazicioglu KM, Doseyen Z, Turkcapar AG, Anadol E. Effect of haemodynamic variables on surgically created arteriovenous fistula flow. *Nephrol Dial Transplant* 1997; 12:1684-1688 (evidence level: B)
17. Beathard GA, Settle SM, Shields MW. Salvage of the nonfunctioning arteriovenous fistula. *Am J Kidney Dis.* 1999; 33: 910-916
18. Turmel-Rodrigues L, Mouton A, Birmele B, Billaux L, Ammar N, Grezard O, Hauss S, Pengloan J. Salvage of immature forearm fistulas for haemodialysis by interventional radiology. *Nephrol Dial Transplant* 2001; 16: 2365-2371
19. Wittenberg G, Schindler T, Tschammler A, Kenn W, Hahn D. [Value of color-coded duplex ultrasound in evaluating arm blood vessels-arteries and hemodialysis shunts]. *Ultraschall Med* 1998; 19:22-27
20. Malovrh M. Native arteriovenous fistula: preoperative evaluation. *Am J Kidney Dis* 2002; 39:1218-1225
21. Wong V, Ward R, Taylor J, Selvakumar S, How TV, Bakran A. Factors associated with early failure of arteriovenous fistulae for haemodialysis access. *Eur J Vasc Endovasc Surg* 1996; 12:207-213 (evidence level: B)
22. Sidawy AN, Gray R, Besarab A, Henry M, Ascher E, Silva M, Jr., Miller A, Scher L, Trerotola S, Gregory RT, Rutherford RB, Kent KC. Recommended standards for reports dealing with arteriovenous hemodialysis accesses. *J Vasc Surg* 2002; 35:603-610
23. Ascher E, Gade P, Hingorani A, Mazzariol F, Gunduz Y, Fodera M, Yorkovich W. Changes in the practice of angioaccess surgery: impact of dialysis outcome and quality initiative recommendations. *J Vasc Surg* 2000; 31:84-92 (evidence level: B)
24. Bagolan P, Spagnoli A, Ciprandi G, Picca S, Leozappa G, Nahom A, Trucchi A, Rizzoni G, Fabbrini G. A ten-year experience of Brescia-Cimino arteriovenous fistula in children: technical evolution and refinements. *J Vasc Surg* 1998; 27:640-644 (evidence level: B)
25. Bourquelot P, Cussenot O, Corbi P, Pillion G, Gagnadoux MF, Bensman A, Loirat C, Broyer M. Microsurgical creation and follow-up of arteriovenous fistulae for chronic haemodialysis in children. *Pediatr Nephrol* 1990; 4:156-159 (evidence level: B)
26. Rieger J, Sitter T, Toepfer M, Linsenmaier U, Pfeifer KJ, Schiffl H. Gadolinium as an alternative contrast agent for diagnostic and interventional angiographic procedures in patients with impaired renal function. *Nephrol Dial Transplant* 2002; 17:824-828

References

27. Geoffroy O, Tassart M, Le Blanche AF, Khalil A, Duedal V, Rossert J, Bigot JM, Boudghene FP. Upper extremity digital subtraction venography with gadoterate meglumine before fistula creation for hemodialysis. *Kidney Int* 2001; 59:1491-1497 (evidence level: B)
28. Nyman U, Elmstahl B, Leander P, Nilsson M, Golman K, Almen T. Are gadolinium-based contrast media really safer than iodinated media for digital subtraction angiography in patients with azotemia? *Radiology* 2002; 223:311-318 (evidence level: C)
29. Menegazzo D, Laissy JP, Durrbach A, Debray MP, Messin B, Delmas V, Mignon F, Schouman-Claeys E. Hemodialysis access fistula creation: preoperative assessment with MR venography and comparison with conventional venography. *Radiology* 1998; 209:723-728 (evidence level: B)
30. Turmel-Rodrigues L., Bourquelot P, Raynaud A., Beyssen B. Hemodialysis fistula: preoperative MR venography. A promising but partial view. *Radiology* 2000; 211:302 (evidence level: C)
31. Rodriguez JA, Armadans L, Ferrer E, Olmos A, Codina S, Bartolome J, Borrellas J, Piera L. The function of permanent vascular access. *Nephrol Dial Transplant* 2000; 15:402-408
32. Turmel-Rodrigues L, Raynaud A, Louail B, Beyssen B, Sapoval M. Manual catheter-directed aspiration and other thrombectomy techniques for declotting native fistulas for hemodialysis. *J Vasc Interv Radiol* 2001; 12:1365-1371 (evidence level: C)
33. Gundry SR, Jones M, Ishihara T, Ferrans VJ. Optimal preparation techniques for human saphenous vein grafts. *Surgery* 1980; 88:785-794
34. Schaeffer U, Tanner B, Strohschneider T, Stadtmuller A, Hannekum A. Damage to arterial and venous endothelial cells in bypass grafts induced by several solutions used in bypass surgery. *Thorac.Cardiovasc.Surg.* 1997; 45:168-171
35. Souza DS, Christofferson RH, Bomfim V, Filbey D. "No-touch" technique using saphenous vein harvested with its surrounding tissue for coronary artery bypass grafting maintains an intact endothelium. *Scand.Cardiovasc.J* 1999; 33:323-329
36. Sayers RD, Watt PA, Muller S, Bell PR, Thurston H. Structural and functional smooth muscle injury after surgical preparation of reversed and non-reversed (in situ) saphenous vein bypass grafts. *Br.J Surg.* 1991; 78:1256-1258
37. Kennedy JH, Lever MJ, Addis BJ, Paneth M. Changes in vein interstitium following distension for aortocoronary bypass. *J Cardiovasc.Surg.(Torino)* 1989; 30:992-995
38. Angelini GD, Breckenridge IM, Psaila JV, Williams HM, Henderson AH, Newby AC. Preparation of human saphenous vein for coronary artery bypass grafting impairs its capacity to produce prostacyclin. *Cardiovasc.Res.* 1987; 21:28-33
39. Bush HL, Jr., Jakubowski JA, Curl GR, Deykin D, Nabseth DC. The natural history of endothelial structure and function in arterialized vein grafts. *J Vasc Surg* 1986; 3:204-215
40. Svendsen E, Dalen H, Moland J, Engedal H. A quantitative study of endothelial cell injury in aorto-coronary vein grafts. *J Cardiovasc Surg* (Torino) 1986; 27:65-71
41. Haudenschild C, Gould KE, Quist WC, LoGerfo FW. Protection of endothelium in vessel segments excised for grafting. *Circulation* 1981; 64:II101-II107
42. Anderson CB, Etheredge EE, Harter HR, Codd JE, Graff RJ, Newton WT. Blood flow measurements in arteriovenous dialysis fistulas. *Surgery* 1977; 81:459-461
43. Reilly DT, Wood RF, Bell PR. Arteriovenous fistulas for dialysis: blood flow, viscosity, and long- term patency. *World J Surg* 1982; 6:628-633 (evidence level: B)

44. Silva MB, Jr., Hobson RW, Pappas PJ, Haser PB, Araki CT, Goldberg MC, Jamil Z, Padberg FT, Jr. Vein transposition in the forearm for autogenous hemodialysis access. *J Vasc Surg* 1997; 26:981-986 (evidence level: B)
45. Konner K. The anastomosis of the arteriovenous fistula-common errors and their avoidance. *Nephrol Dial Transplant* 2002; 17:376-379 (evidence level: C)

References – Placement of Elbow or Upper Arm A/V Fistula

---

1. Konner K. Primary vascular access in diabetic patients: an audit. *Nephrol Dial Transplant* 2000; 15:1317-1325 (evidence level: B)
2. Hakaim AG, Nalbandian M, Scott T. Superior maturation and patency of primary brachiocephalic and transposed basilic vein arteriovenous fistulae in patients with diabetes. *J Vasc Surg* 1998; 27:154-157 (evidence level: B)
3. Kinnaert P, Vereerstraeten P, Toussaint C, Van Geertruyden J. Nine years' experience with internal arteriovenous fistulas for haemodialysis: a study of some factors influencing the results. *Br J Surg*. 1977; 64: 242-246
4. Rodriguez JA, Armadans L, Ferrer E, Olmos A, Codina S, Bartolome J, Borrellas J, Piera L. The function of permanent vascular access. *Nephrol Dial Transplant.* 2000; 15: 402-408
5. Dixon BS, Novak L, Fangman J. Hemodialysis vascular access survival: Upper-arm native arteriovenous fistula. *Am J Kidney Dis* 2002; 39:92-101 (evidence level: B)
6. Mihmanli I, Besirli K, Kurugoglu S, Atakir K, Haider S, Ogut G, Numan F, Canturk E, Sayin AG. Cephalic vein and hemodialysis fistula: surgeon's observation versus color Doppler ultrasonographic findings. *J Ultrasound Med* 2001; 20:217-222 (evidence level: A)
7. Rubens F and Wellington JL. Brachiocephalic fistula: a useful alternative for vascular access in chronic hemodialysis. *Cardiovasc Surg* 1993; 1:128-130 (evidence level: B)
8. Young PR, Jr., Rohr MS, Marterre WF, Jr. High-output cardiac failure secondary to a brachiocephalic arteriovenous hemodialysis fistula: two cases. *Am Surg* 1998; 64:239-241 (evidence level: B)
9. Schenk WG, III. Subclavian steal syndrome from high-output brachiocephalic arteriovenous fistula: a previously undescribed complication of dialysis access. *J Vasc Surg* 2001; 33:883-885 (evidence level: B)
10. Yerdel MA, Kesenci M, Yazicioglu KM, Doseyen Z, Turkcapar AG, Anadol E. Effect of haemodynamic variables on surgically created arteriovenous fistula flow. *Nephrol Dial Transplant* 1997; 12:1684-1688 (evidence level: B)
11. Ascher E, Gade P, Hingorani A, Mazzariol F, Gunduz Y, Fodera M, Yorkovich W. Changes in the practice of angioaccess surgery: impact of dialysis outcome and quality initiative recommendations. *J Vasc Surg* 2000; 31:84-92 (evidence level: B)
12. Dagher F, Gelber R, Ramos E, Sadler J. The use of basilic vein and brachial artery as an A-V fistula for long term hemodialysis. *J Surg Res* 1976; 20:373-376 (evidence level: B)
13. Elcheroth J, de Pauw L, Kinnaert P. Elbow arteriovenous fistulas for chronic haemodialysis. *Br J Surg* 1994; 81:982-984 (evidence level: B)
14. Rivers SP, Scher LA, Sheehan E, Lynn R, Veith FJ. Basilic vein transposition: an underused autologous alternative to prosthetic dialysis angioaccess. *J Vasc Surg* 1993; 18:391-396 (evidence level: B)

15. Hibberd AD. Brachiobasilic fistula with autogenous basilic vein: surgical technique and pilot study. *Aust N Z J Surg* 1991; 61:631-635 (evidence level: B)
16. Burkhart HM and Cikrit DF. Arteriovenous fistulae for hemodialysis. *Semin Vasc Surg* 1997; 10:162-165 (evidence level: C)
17. Oliver MJ, McCann RL, Indridason OS, Butterly DW, Schwab SJ. Comparison of transposed brachiobasilic fistulas to upper arm grafts and brachiocephalic fistulas. *Kidney Int* 2001; 60:1532-1539 (evidence level: B)
18. Murphy GJ, White SA, Knight AJ, Doughman T, Nicholson ML. Long-term results of arteriovenous fistulas using transposed autologous basilic vein. *Br J Surg* 2000; 87:819-823 (evidence level: B)
19. Polo JR, Vazquez R, Polo J, Sanabia J, Rueda JA, Lopez-Baena JA. Brachiocephalic jump graft fistula: an alternative for dialysis use of elbow crease veins. *Am J Kidney Dis* 1999; 33:904-909 (evidence level: B)

References – Placement of Graft

1. Tordoir JH, Kwan TS, Herman JM, Carol EJ, Jakimowicz JJ. Primary and secondary access surgery for haemodialysis with the Brescia- Cimino fistula and the polytetrafluoroethylene (PTFE) graft. *Neth J Surg* 1983; 35:8-12 (evidence level: B)
2. Fong IW, Capellan JM, Simbul M, Angel J. Infection of arterio-venous fistulas created for chronic haemodialysis. *Scand J Infect Dis* 1993; 25:215-220 (evidence level: B)
3. Nassar GM and Ayus JC. Infectious complications of the hemodialysis access. *Kidney Int* 2001; 60:1-13 (evidence level: C)
4. Ascher E, Gade P, Hingorani A, Mazzariol F, Gunduz Y, Fodera M, Yorkovich W. Changes in the practice of angioaccess surgery: impact of dialysis outcome and quality initiative recommendations. *J Vasc Surg* 2000; 31:84-92 (evidence level: B)
5. Turmel-Rodrigues L, Pengloan J, Baudin S, Testou D, Abaza M, Dahdah G, Mouton A, Blanchard D. Treatment of stenosis and thrombosis in haemodialysis fistulas and grafts by interventional radiology. *Nephrol Dial Transplant* 2000; 15:2029-2036 (evidence level: B)
6. Ruddle AC, Lear PA, Mitchell DC. The morbidity of secondary vascular access. A lifetime of intervention. Eur J Vasc Endovasc Surg 1999; 18:30-34 (evidence level: B)
7. Murray BM, Rajczak S, Ali B, Herman A, Mepani B. Assessment of access blood flow after preemptive angioplasty. *Am J Kidney Dis* 2001; 37:1029-1038 (evidence level: B)
8. Smits JH, van der Linden J, Hagen EC, Modderkolk-Cammeraat EC, Feith GW, Koomans HA, van den Dorpel MA, Blankestijn PJ. Graft surveillance: venous pressure, access flow, or the combination? *Kidney Int* 2001; 59:1551-1558 (evidence level: A)
9. Dhingra RK, Young EW, Hulbert-Shearon TE, Leavey SF, Port FK. Type of vascular access and mortality in U.S. hemodialysis patients. *Kidney Int* 2001; 60:1443-1451 (evidence level: B)
10. Staramos DN, Lazarides MK, Tzilalis VD, Ekonomou CS, Simopoulos CE, Dayantas JN. Patency of autologous and prosthetic arteriovenous fistulas in elderly patients. *Eur J Surg* 2000; 166:777-781 (evidence level: B)

11. Lemson MS, Tordoir JH, van Det RJ, Welten RJ, Burger H, Estourgie RJ, Stroecken HJ, Leunissen KM. Effects of a venous cuff at the venous anastomosis of polytetrafluoroethylene grafts for hemodialysis vascular access. *J Vasc Surg* 2000; 32:1155-1163 (evidence level: A)
12. Tordoir JH, Hofstra L, Leunissen KM, Kitslaar PJ. Early experience with stretch polytetrafluoroethylene grafts for haemodialysis access surgery: results of a prospective randomised study. Eur J Vasc Endovasc Surg 1995; 9:305-309 (evidence level: A)
13. Silva MB, Jr., Hobson RW, Pappas PJ, Jamil Z, Araki CT, Goldberg MC, Gwertzman G, Padberg FT, Jr. A strategy for increasing use of autogenous hemodialysis access procedures: impact of preoperative noninvasive evaluation. *J Vasc Surg* 1998; 27:302-307 (evidence level: B)
14. Lazarides MK, Iatrou CE, Karanikas ID, Kaperonis NM, Petras DI, Zirogiannis PN, Dayantas JN. Factors affecting the lifespan of autologous and synthetic arteriovenous access routes for haemodialysis. *Eur J Surg* 1996; 162:297-301 (evidence level: D)
15. Dracon M, Watine O, Pruvot F, Noel C, Lelievre G. [Axillo-axillary access in hemodialysis]. *Nephrologie* 1994; 15:175-176 (evidence level: B)
16. Ono K, Muto Y, Yano K, Yukizane T. Anterior chest wall axillary artery to contralateral axillary vein graft for vascular access in hemodialysis. *Artif Organs* 1995; 19:1233-1236 (evidence level: B)
17. Polo JR, Sanabia J, Garcia-Sabrido JL, Luno J, Menarguez C, Echenagusia A. Brachial-jugular polytetrafluoroethylene fistulas for hemodialysis. *Am J Kidney Dis* 1990; 16:465-468 (evidence level: B)
18. Vega D, Polo JR, Polo J, Lopez Baena JA, Pacheco D, Garcia-Pajares R. Brachial-jugular expanded PTFE grafts for dialysis. *Ann Vasc Surg* 2001; 15:553-556
19. Allon M, Bailey R, Ballard R, Deierhoi MH, Hamrick K, Oser R, Rhynes VK, Robbin ML, Saddekni S, Zeigler ST. A multidisciplinary approach to hemodialysis access: prospective evaluation. *Kidney Int* 1998; 53:473-479 (evidence level: B)
20. Polo JR, Tejedor A, Polo J, Sanabia J, Calleja J, Gomez F. Long-term follow-up of 6-8 mm brachioaxillary polytetrafluoroethylene grafts for hemodialysis. *Artif Organs* 1995; 19:1181-1184 (evidence level B)
21. Barron PT, Wellington JL, Lorimer JW, Cole CW, Moher D. A comparison between expanded polytetrafluoroethylene and plasma tetrafluoroethylene grafts for hemodialysis access. *Can J Surg* 1993; 36:184-186 (evidence level: A-B)
22. Helling TS, Nelson PW, Shelton L. A prospective evaluation of plasma-TFE and expanded PTFE grafts for routine and early use as vascular access during hemodialysis. *Ann Surg* 1992; 216:596-599 (evidence level: A-B)
23. Nakagawa Y, Ota K, Sato Y, Teraoka S, Agishi T. Clinical trial of new polyurethane vascular grafts for hemodialysis: compared with expanded polytetrafluoroethylene grafts. *Artif Organs* 1995; 19:1227-1232 (evidence level: B)
24. Lenz BJ, Veldenz HC, Dennis JW, Khansarinia S, Atteberry LR. A three-year follow-up on standard versus thin wall ePTFE grafts for hemodialysis. *J Vasc Surg* 1998; 28:464-470 (evidence level: A)
25. Zibari GB, Gadallah MF, Landreneau M, McMillan R, Bridges RM, Costley K, Work J, McDonald JC. Preoperative vancomycin prophylaxis decreases incidence of postoperative hemodialysis vascular access infections. *Am J Kidney Dis* 1997; 30:343-348 (evidence level: A)
26. Polo J. (personnel communication)

27. Korzets A, Ori Y, Baytner S, Zevin D, Chagnac A, Weinstein T, Herman M, Agmon M, Gafter U. The femoral artery-femoral vein polytetrafluoroethylene graft: a 14- year retrospective study. *Nephrol Dial Transplant* 1998; 13:1215-1220 (evidence level: B)
28. Gradman WS, Cohen W, Haji-Aghaii M. Arteriovenous fistula construction in the thigh with transposed superficial femoral vein: our initial experience. *J Vasc Surg* 2001; 33:968-975 (evidence level: B)

References – Placement and Routine Management of Tunneled Catheter

1. Canaud B, My H, Morena M, Lamy-Lacavalerie B, Leray-Moragues H, Bosc JY, Flavier JL, Chomel PY, Polaschegg HD, Prosl FR, Megerman J. Dialock: a new vascular access device for extracorporeal renal replacement therapy. Preliminary clinical results. *Nephrol Dial Transplant* 1999; 14:692-698 (evidence level: B)
2. Kessler M, Canaud B, Pedrini MT, Tattersall JE, ter Wee PM, Vanholder R, Wanner C. European Best Practice Guidelines for Haemodialysis (Part 1). *Nephrol Dial Transplant* 2002; 17 (Suppl. 7)
3. Work J. Chronic catheter placement. *Semin Dial* 2001; 14:436-440 (evidence level: C)
4. Oliver MJ. Acute dialysis catheters. *Semin Dial* 2001; 14:432-435 (evidence level: C)
5. Cimochowski GE, Worley E, Rutherford WE, Sartain J, Blondin J, Harter H. Superiority of the internal jugular over the subclavian access for temporary dialysis. *Nephron* 1990; 54:154-161 (evidence level: B)
6. Schillinger F, Schillinger D, Montagnac R, Milcent T. Post catheterisation vein stenosis in haemodialysis: comparative angiographic study of 50 subclavian and 50 internal jugular accesses. *Nephrol Dial Transplant* 1991; 6:722-724 (evidence level: B)
7. Trerotola SO, Kuhn-Fulton J, Johnson MS, Shah H, Ambrosius WT, Kneebone PH. Tunneled infusion catheters: increased incidence of symptomatic venous thrombosis after subclavian versus internal jugular venous access. *Radiology* 2000; 217:89-93 (evidence level: B)
8. Jean G, Vanel T, Chazot C et al. [Prevalence of stenosis and thrombosis of central veins in hemodialysis after a tunneled jugular catheter]. *Nephrologie* 2001; 22: 501-504
9. Zaleski GX, Funaki B, Lorenz JM, Garofalo RS, Moscatel MA, Rosenblum JD, Leef JA. Experience with tunneled femoral hemodialysis catheters. *Am J Roentgenol* 1999; 172:493-496 (evidence level: B)
10. Webb A, Abdalla M, Harden PN, Russell GI. Use of the Tesio catheter for hemodialysis in patients with end-stage renal failure: a 2-year prospective study. *Clin Nephrol* 2002; 58: 128-133
11. Chow KM, Szeto CC, Leung CB, Wong TY, Li PK. Cuffed-tunneled femoral catheter for long-term hemodialysis. *Int J Artif Organs* 2001; 24: 443-446
12. Trerotola SO, Shah H, Johnson M, Namyslowski J, Moresco K, Patel N, Kraus M, Gassensmith C, Ambrosius WT. Randomized comparison of high-flow versus conventional hemodialysis catheters. *J Vasc Interv Radiol* 1999; 10:1032-1038 (evidence level: A)
13. Schwab SJ and Beathard G. The hemodialysis catheter conundrum: hate living with them, but can't live without them. *Kidney Int* 1999; 56:1-17 (evidence level: C)
14. Depner TA. Catheter performance. *Semin Dial* 2001; 14:425-431 (evidence level: C)

15. Twardowski ZJ and Seger RM. Dimensions of central venous structures in humans measured in vivo using magnetic resonance imaging: implications for central-vein catheter dimensions. *Int J Artif Organs* 2002; 25:107-123 (evidence level: C)
16. Leblanc M, Fedak S, Mokris G, Paganini EP. Blood recirculation in temporary central catheters for acute hemodialysis. *Clin Nephrol* 1996; 45:315-319
17. Little MA, Conlon PJ, Walshe JJ. Access recirculation in temporary hemodialysis catheters as measured by the saline dilution technique. *Am J Kidney Dis* 2000; 36:1135-1139 (evidence level: B)
18. Denys BG, Uretsky BF, Reddy PS. Ultrasound-assisted cannulation of the internal jugular vein. A prospective comparison to the external landmark-guided technique. *Circulation* 1993; 87:1557-1562 (evidence level: A)
19. Teichgraber UK, Benter T, Gebel M, Manns MP. A sonographically guided technique for central venous access. *AJR Am J Roentgenol* 1997; 169:731-733 (evidence level: A)
20. Iseng M, Sadler D, Wong J, Teague KR, Schemmer DC, Saliken JC, So B, Gray RR Radiologic placement of central venous catheters: rates of success and immediate complications in 3412 cases. *Can Assoc Radiol J* 2001; 52:379-384 (evidence level: B)
21. Kwon TH, Kim YL, Cho DK. Ultrasound-guided cannulation of the femoral vein for acute haemodialysis access. *Nephrol Dial Transplant* 1997; 12:1009-1012
22. Petersen J, Delaney JH, Brakstad MT, Rowbotham RK, Bagley CM, Jr. Silicone venous access devices positioned with their tips high in the superior vena cava are more likely to malfunction. *Am J Surg* 1999; 178:38-41 (evidence level: B)
23. Jean G, Chazot C, Vanel T, Charra B, Terrat JC, Calemard E, Laurent G. Central venous catheters for haemodialysis: looking for optimal blood flow. *Nephrol Dial Transplant* 1997; 12:1689-1691 (evidence level: B)
24. Conly JM, Grieves K, Peters B. A prospective, randomized study comparing transparent and dry gauze dressings for central venous catheters. *J Infect Dis* 1989; 159:310-319 (evidence level: A)
25. Levin A, Mason AJ, Jindal KK, Fong IW, Goldstein MB. Prevention of hemodialysis subclavian vein catheter infections by topical povidone-iodine. *Kidney Int* 1991; 40:934-938 (evidence level: A)
26. Ash SR. The evolution and function of central venous catheters for dialysis. *Semin Dial* 2001; 14:416-424 (evidence level: C)
27. Kairaitis LK and Gottlieb T. Outcome and complications of temporary haemodialysis catheters. *Nephrol Dial Transplant* 1999; 14:1710-1714 (evidence level: B)
28. Karaaslan H, Peyronnet P, Benevent D, Lagarde C, Rince M, Leroux-Robert C. Risk of heparin lock-related bleeding when using indwelling venous catheter in haemodialysis. Nephrol Dial Transplant 2001; 16:2072-2074 (evidence level: B)
29. Trivedi HS and Twardowski ZJ. Use of double-lumen dialysis catheters. Loading with locked heparin. *ASAIO J* 1997; 43:900-903 (evidence level: B)
30. Buturovic J, Ponikvar R, Kandus A, Boh M, Klinkmann J, Ivanovich P. Filling hemodialysis catheters in the interdialytic period: heparin versus citrate versus polygeline: a prospective randomized study. *Artif Organs* 1998; 22:945-947 (evidence level: B)
31. Stas KJ, Vanwalleghem J, De Moor B, Keuleers H. Trisodium citrate 30 % vs. heparin 5 % as catheter lock in the interdialytic period in. *Nephrol Dial Transplant* 2001; 16:1521-1522 (evidence level: B)

32. Quarello F and Forneris G. Prevention of hemodialysis catheter-related bloodstream infection using an antimicrobial lock. *Blood Purif* 2002; 20:87-92 (evidence level: B)
33. Vercaigne LM, Sitar DS, Penner SB, Bernstein K, Wang GQ, Burczynski FJ. Antibiotic-heparin lock: in vitro antibiotic stability combined with heparin in a central venous catheter. *Pharmacotherapy* 2000; 20:394-399 (evidence level: B)
34. Ash S. Concentrated Sodium Citrate as Catheter Lock Solution. *J Am Soc Nephrol* 1999; 10:272 (evidence level: B)
35. Yu VL, Goetz A, Wagener M, Smith PB, Rihs JD, Hanchett J, Zuravleff JJ. Staphylococcus aureus nasal carriage and infection in patients on hemodialysis. Efficacy of antibiotic prophylaxis. *N Engl J Med* 1986; 315:91-96 (evidence level: A)
36. Koziol-Montewka M, Chudnicka A, Ksiazek A, Majdan M. Rate of Staphylococcus aureus nasal carriage in immunocompromised patients receiving haemodialysis treatment. *Int J Antimicrob Agents* 2001; 18:193-196 (evidence level: B)
37. Piraino B. Staphylococcus aureus infections in dialysis patients: focus on prevention. *ASAIO J* 2000; 46:S13-S17 (evidence level: B)
38. Level C, Lasseur C, Chauveau P, Bonarek H, Perrault L, Combe C. Performance of twin central venous catheters: influence of the inversion of inlet and outlet on recirculation. *Blood Purif* 2002; 20:182-188 (evidence level: B)

References – Postoperative Control of A/V Fistula and Graft Function (1)

1. III. NKF-K/DOQI Clinical Practice Guidelines for Vascular Access: update 2000. *Am J Kidney Dis* 2001; 37 (Suppl. 1) :S137-S181
2. Palder SB, Kirkman RL, Whittemore AD, Hakim RM, Lazarus JM, Tilney NL. Vascular access for hemodialysis. Patency rates and results of revision. *Ann Surg* 1985; 202:235-239 (evidence level: B)
3. Nicholson ML and Murphy GJ Surgical considerations in vascular access. New York, Oxford University Press 2000; 101-123 (evidence level: C)
4. Deneuville M. Infection of PTFE grafts used to create arteriovenous fistulas for hemodialysis access. *Ann Vasc Surg* 2000; 14:473-479 (evidence level: B)
5. Nghiem DD, Schulak JA, Corry RJ. Management of the infected hemodialysis access grafts. *Trans Am Soc Artif Intern Organs* 1983; 29:360-362 (evidence level: B)
6. Padberg FT, Jr., Lee BC, Curl GR. Hemoaccess site infection. *Surg Gynecol Obstet* 1992; 174:103-108 (evidence level: B)

References – Postoperative Control of A/V Fistula and Graft Function (2)

1. Tautenhahn J, Heinrich P, Meyer F. [Arteriovenous fistulas for hemodialysis-patency rates and complications--a retrospective study]. *Zentralbl Chir* 1994; 119:506-510 (evidence level: B)
2. Bay WH, Van Cleef S, Owens M. The hemodialysis access: preferences and concerns of patients, dialysis nurses and technicians, and physicians. *Am J Nephrol* 1998; 18:379-383 (evidence level: B)
3. Yerdel MA, Kesenci M, Yazicioglu KM, Doseyen Z, Turkcapar AG, Anadol E. Effect of haemodynamic variables on surgically created arteriovenous fistula flow. *Nephrol Dial Transplant* 1997; 12:1684-1688 (evidence level: B)

4. Sivanesan S, How TV, Bakran A. Characterizing flow distributions in AV fistulae for haemodialysis access. *Nephrol Dial Transplant* 1998; 13:3108-3110 (evidence level: B)
5. Turmel-Rodrigues L, Mouton A, Birmele B, Billaux L, Ammar N, Grezard O, Hauss S, Pengloan J. Salvage of immature forearm fistulas for haemodialysis by interventional radiology. *Nephrol Dial Transplant* 2001; 16:2365-2371 (evidence level: B)
6. Faiyaz R, Abreo K, Zaman F, Pervez A, Zibari G, Work J. Salvage of poorly developed arteriovenous fistulae with percutaneous ligation of accessory veins. *Am J Kidney Dis* 2002; 39:824-827 (evidence level: B)
7. Konner K, Hulbert-Shearon TE, Roys EC, Port FK. Tailoring the initial vascular access for dialysis patients. *Kidney Int* 2002; 62:329-338 (evidence level: B)
8. Jindal KK, Ethier JH, Lindsay RM, Barre PE, Kappel JE, Carlisle EJ, Common A. Clinical practice guidelines for vascular access. Canadian Society of Nephrology. *J Am Soc Nephrol* 1999; 10 Suppl 13:S297-S305 (evidence level: C)
9. Kessler M, Canaud B, Pedrini MT, Tattersall JE, ter Wee P.M., Vanholder R, Wanner C. European Best Practice Guidelines for Haemodialysis (Part 1). *Nephrol Dial Transplant* 2002; 17 (Suppl. 7)
10. Koksoy C, Kuzu A, Erden I, Turkcapar AG, Duzgun I, Anadol E. Predictive value of colour Doppler ultrasonography in detecting failure of vascular access grafts. *Br J Surg* 1995; 82:50-52
11. Wong V, Ward R, Taylor J, Selvakumar S, How TV, Bakran A. Factors associated with early failure of arteriovenous fistulae for haemodialysis access. *Eur J Vasc Endovasc Surg* 1996; 12:207-213 (evidence level: B)
12. Lin SL, Chen HS, Huang CH, Yen TS. Predicting the outcome of hemodialysis arteriovenous fistulae using duplex ultrasonography. *J Formos Med Assoc* 1997; 96:864-868 (evidence level: B)
13. Turmel-Rodrigues L, Raynaud A, Bourquelot P. Percutaneous treatment of arteriovenous access dysfunction. Oxford, *New York Oxford University Press* 2000; 183-202 (evidence level: C)
14. Konner K. Interventional strategies for haemodialysis fistulae and grafts: interventional radiology or surgery? *Nephrol Dial Transplant* 2000; 15:1922-1923 (evidence level: C)

References – Routine Management of A/V Fistula and Graft

1. Nassar GM and Ayus JC. Infectious complications of the hemodialysis access. *Kidney Int* 2001; 60:1-13 (evidence level: C)
2. Trerotola SO, Scheel PJ, Jr., Powe NR, Prescott C, Feeley N, He J, Watson A. Screening for dialysis access graft malfunction: comparison of physical examination with US. *J Vasc Interv Radiol* 1996; 7:15-20 (evidence level: B)
3. Lazarides MK, Staramos DN, Panagopoulos GN, Tzilalis VD, Eleftheriou GJ, Dayantas JN, Staamos DN. Indications for surgical treatment of angioaccess-induced arterial "steal". *J Am Coll Surg* 1998; 187:422-426 (evidence level: B)
4. Miles AM. Upper limb ischemia after vascular access surgery: differential diagnosis and management. *Semin Dial* 2000; 13:312-315 (evidence level: C)

5. Gallego Beuter JJ, Hernandez LA, Herrero CJ, Moreno CR. Early detection and treatment of hemodialysis access dysfunction. *Cardiovasc Intervent Radiol* 2000; 23:40-46 (evidence level: B)
6. Depner TA, Krivitski NM, MacGibbon D. Hemodialysis access recirculation measured by ultrasound dilution. *ASAIO J* 1995; 41:M749-M753 (evidence level: B)
7. Sands J, Young S, Miranda C. The effect of Doppler flow screening studies and elective revisions on dialysis access failure. *ASAIO J* 1992; 38:M524-M527 (evidence level: B)
8. May RE, Himmelfarb J, Yenicesu M, Knights S, Ikizler TA, Schulman G, Hernanz-Schulman M, Shyr Y, Hakim RM. Predictive measures of vascular access thrombosis: a prospective study. *Kidney Int* 1997; 52:1656-1662 (evidence level: B)
9. Bosman PJ, Boereboom FT, Eikelboom BC, Koomans HA, Blankestijn PJ. Graft flow as a predictor of thrombosis in hemodialysis grafts. *Kidney Int* 1998; 54:1726-1730 (evidence level: B)
10. Besarab A. Intervention for intra-access stenosis. *Semin Dial* 2001; 14:401-402 (evidence level: C)
11. McDougal G and Agarwal R. Clinical performance characteristics of hemodialysis graft monitoring. *Kidney Int* 2001; 60:762-766 (evidence level: B)
12. Schwab SJ, Raymond JR, Saeed M, Newman GE, Dennis PA, Bollinger RR. Prevention of hemodialysis fistula thrombosis. Early detection of venous stenoses. *Kidney Int* 1989; 36:707-711 (evidence level: B)
13. Depner TA, Rizwan S, Stasi TA. Pressure effects on roller pump blood flow during hemodialysis. *ASAIO Trans* 1990; 36:M456-M459 (evidence level: B)
14. Francos GC, Burke JF, Jr., Besarab A, Martinez J, Kirkwood RG, Hummel LA. An unsuspected cause of acute hemolysis during hemodialysis. *Trans Am Soc Artif Intern Organs* 1983; 29:140-145 (evidence level: B)
15. Sands J. The role of color-flow Doppler ultrasound in the management of hemodialysis accesses. *ASAIO J* 1998; 44:41-43 (evidence level: C)
16. Smits JH, van der Linden J, Hagen EC, Modderkolk-Cammeraat EC, Feith GW, Koomans HA, van den Dorpel MA, Blankestijn PJ. Graft surveillance: venous pressure, access flow, or the combination? *Kidney Int* 2001; 59:1551-1558 (evidence level: A)
17. Schwab SJ, Oliver MJ, Suhocki P, McCann R. Hemodialysis arteriovenous access: detection of stenosis and response to treatment by vascular access blood flow. *Kidney Int* 2001; 59:358-362 (evidence level: B)
18. Sands JJ, Jabyac PA, Miranda CL, Kapsick BJ. Intervention based on monthly monitoring decreases hemodialysis access thrombosis. *ASAIO J* 1999; 45:147-150 (evidence level: A)
19. Beathard GA. Percutaneous transvenous angioplasty in the treatment of vascular access stenosis. *Kidney Int* 1992; 42:1390-1397 (evidence level: B)
20. III. NKF-K/DOQI Clinical Practice Guidelines for Vascular Access: update 2000. *Am J Kidney Dis* 2001; 37 (Suppl. 1) : S137-S181
21. Tonelli M, Jindal K, Hirsch D, Taylor S, Kane C, Henbrey S. Screening for subclinical stenosis in native vessel arteriovenous fistulae. *J Am Soc Nephrol* 2001; 12:1729-1733 (evidence level: B)
22. Weitzel WF, Khosla N, Rubin JM. Retrograde hemodialysis access flow during dialysis as a predictor of access pathology. *Am J Kidney Dis* 2001; 37:1241-1246 (evidence level: B)

23. Neyra NR, Ikizler TA, May RE, Himmelfarb J, Schulman G, Shyr Y, Hakim RM. Change in access blood flow over time predicts vascular access thrombosis. *Kidney Int* 1998; 54:1714-1719 (evidence level: B)
24. McCarley P, Wingard RL, Shyr Y, Pettus W, Hakim RM, Ikizler TA. Vascular access blood flow monitoring reduces access morbidity and costs. *Kidney Int* 2001; 60:1164-1172 (evidence level: B)
25. Lindsay RM, Bradfield E, Rothera C, Kianfar C, Malek P, Blake PG. A comparison of methods for the measurement of hemodialysis access recirculation and access blood flow rate. *ASAIO J* 1998; 44:62-67 (evidence level: C)
26. Lindsay RM, Blake PG, Malek P, Posen G, Martin B, Bradfield E. Hemodialysis access blood flow rates can be measured by a differential conductivity technique and are predictive of access clotting. *Am J Kidney Dis* 1997; 30:475-482 (evidence level: B)
27. Steuer RR, Miller DR, Zhang S, Bell DA, Leypoldt JK. Noninvasive transcutaneous determination of access blood flow rate. *Kidney Int* 2001; 60:284-291 (evidence level: B)
28. Schneditz D, Wang E, Levin NW. Validation of haemodialysis recirculation and access blood flow measured by thermodilution. *Nephrol Dial Transplant* 1999; 14:376-383 (evidence level: B)
29. Rehman SU, Pupim LB, Shyr Y, Hakim R, Ikizler TA. Intradialytic serial vascular access flow measurements. *Am J Kidney Dis* 1999; 34:471-477 (evidence level: B)
30. Agharazii M, Clouatre Y, Nolin L, Leblanc M. Variation of intra-access flow early and late into hemodialysis. *ASAIO J* 2000; 46:452-455 (evidence level: B)
31. Jindal KK, Ethier JH, Lindsay RM, Barre PE, Kappel JE, Carlisle EJ, Common A. Clinical practice guidelines for vascular access. Canadian Society of Nephrology. *J Am Soc Nephrol* 1999; 10 Suppl 13:S297-S305 (evidence level: C)
32. Paulson WD, Ram SJ, Birk CG, Work J. Does blood flow accurately predict thrombosis or failure of hemodialysis synthetic grafts? A meta-analysis. *Am J Kidney Dis* 1999; 34:478-485 (evidence level: B)
33. Paulson WD, Ram SJ, Birk CG, Zapczynski M, Martin SR, Work J. Accuracy of decrease in blood flow in predicting hemodialysis graft thrombosis. *Am J Kidney Dis* 2000; 35:1089-1095 (evidence level: B)
34. Wang E, Schneditz D, Nepomuceno C, Lavarias V, Martin K, Morris AT, Levin NW. Predictive value of access blood flow in detecting access thrombosis. *ASAIO J* 1998; 44:M555-M558 (evidence level: B)
35. Lumsden AB, MacDonald MJ, Kikeri D, Cotsonis GA, Harker LA, Martin LG. Cost efficacy of duplex surveillance and prophylactic angioplasty of arteriovenous ePTFE grafts. *Ann Vasc Surg* 1998; 12:138-142 (evidence level: A-B)
36. Besarab A, Sullivan KL, Ross RP, Moritz MJ. Utility of intra-access pressure monitoring in detecting and correcting venous outlet stenoses prior to thrombosis. *Kidney Int* 1995; 47:1364-1373 (evidence level: B)
37. Dember LM, Holmberg EF, Kaufman JS. Value of static venous pressure for predicting arteriovenous graft thrombosis. *Kidney Int* 2002; 61:1899-1904 (evidence level: B)
38. Kessler M, Canaud B, Pedrini MT, Tattersall JE, ter Wee P.M., Vanholder R, Wanner C. European Best Practice Guidelines for Haemodialysis (Part 1). *Nephrol Dial Transplant* 2002; 17 (Suppl. 7)
39. Krönung G. Aspekte zur Punktion von Dialysezugängen. In: Dialyseshunts: Grund-

lagen, Chirurgie, Komplikationen. Hepp W, Hegenscheid M. (eds), Darmstadt Steinkopf 1998; 241-251 (evidence level: C)
40. Twardowski ZJ. Constant Site (Buttonhole) Method of Needle Insertion for Hemodialysis. *Dialysis & Transplantation* 1995; 24:559-560-576 (evidence level: C)
41. Twardowski ZJ and Kubara H. Different Sites Versus Constant Sites of Needle Insertion Into Arteriovenous Fistulas for Treatment by Repeated Dialysis. *Dialysis & Transplantation* 1979; 8:978-980 (evidence level: B)
42. Boelaert JR, Van Landuyt HW, Godard CA, Daneels RF, Schurgers ML, Matthys EG, De Baere YA, Gheyle DW, Gordts BZ, Herwaldt LA. Nasal mupirocin ointment decreases the incidence of Staphylococcus aureus bacteraemias in haemodialysis patients. *Nephrol Dial Transplant* 1993; 8:235-239 (evidence level: B)

References – Identification of A/V Fistula and Graft Problems

---

1. Trerotola SO, Scheel PJ, Jr., Powe NR, Prescott C, Feeley N, He J, Watson A. Screening for dialysis access graft malfunction: comparison of physical examination with US. *J Vasc Interv Radiol* 1996; 7:15-20 (evidence level: B)
2. Pourchez T. Clinical Diagnosis of Arteriovenous Fistulae Stenosis. *Dialyse-Journal* 1999; 66:232-234 (evidence level: C)
3. Weitzel WF, Khosla N, Rubin JM. Retrograde hemodialysis access flow during dialysis as a predictor of access pathology. *Am J Kidney Dis* 2001; 37:1241-1246 (evidence level: B)
4. Sands J, Young S, Miranda C. The effect of Doppler flow screening studies and elective revisions on dialysis access failure. *ASAIO J* 1992; 38:M524-M527 (evidence level: B)
5. May RE, Himmelfarb J, Yenicesu M, Knights S, Ikizler TA, Schulman G, Hernanz-Schulman M, Shyr Y, Hakim RM. Predictive measures of vascular access thrombosis: a prospective study. *Kidney Int* 1997; 52:1656-1662 (evidence level: B)
6. Lindsay RM, Blake PG, Malek P, Posen G, Martin B, Bradfield E. Hemodialysis access blood flow rates can be measured by a differential conductivity technique and are predictive of access clotting. *Am J Kidney Dis* 1997; 30:475-482 (evidence level: B)
7. Depner TA. Hemodialysis access-the role of monitoring. In-line methods. *ASAIO J* 1998; 44:38-39 (evidence level: C)
8. Bosman PJ, Boereboom FT, Eikelboom BC, Koomans HA, Blankestijn PJ. Graft flow as a predictor of thrombosis in hemodialysis grafts. *Kidney Int* 1998; 54:1726-1730 (evidence level: B)
9. Wang E, Schneditz D, Nepomuceno C, Lavarias V, Martin K, Morris AT, Levin NW. Predictive value of access blood flow in detecting access thrombosis. *ASAIO J* 1998; 44:M555-M558 (evidence level: B)
10. Tonelli M, Jindal K, Hirsch D, Taylor S, Kane C, Henbrey S. Screening for subclinical stenosis in native vessel arteriovenous fistulae. *J Am Soc Nephrol* 2001; 12:1729-1733 (evidence level: B)
11. Jindal KK, Ethier JH, Lindsay RM, Barre PE, Kappel JE, Carlisle EJ, Common A. Clinical practice guidelines for vascular access. Canadian Society of Nephrology. *J Am Soc Nephrol* 1999; 10 Suppl 13:S297-S305 (evidence level: C)
12. Vanholder R. Vascular access: care and monitoring of function. *Nephrol Dial Transplant* 2001; 16:1542-1545 (evidence level: C)

13. Paulson WD, Ram SJ, Birk CG, Work J. Does blood flow accurately predict thrombosis or failure of hemodialysis synthetic grafts? A meta-analysis. *Am J Kidney Dis* 1999; 34: 478-485
14. Neyra NR, Ikizler TA, May RE et al. Change in access blood flow over time predicts vascular access thrombosis. *Kidney Int* 1998; 54: 1714-1719
15. III. NKF-K/DOQI Clinical Practice Guidelines for Vascular Access: update 2000. *Am J Kidney Dis* 2001; 37:S137-S181
16. Gallego Beuter JJ, Hernandez LA, Herrero CJ, Moreno CR. Early detection and treatment of hemodialysis access dysfunction. *Cardiovasc Intervent Radiol* 2000; 23:40-46 (evidence level: B)
17. Schwab SJ, Oliver MJ, Suhocki P, McCann R. Hemodialysis arteriovenous access: detection of stenosis and response to treatment by vascular access blood flow. *Kidney Int* 2001; 59:358-362 (evidence level: B)
18. Paulson WD, Ram SJ, Birk CG, Work J. Does blood flow accurately predict thrombosis or failure of hemodialysis synthetic grafts? A meta-analysis. *Am J Kidney Dis* 1999; 34:478-485 (evidence level: B)
19. Greenwood RN, Aldridge C, Goldstein L, Baker LR, Cattell WR. Assessment of arteriovenous fistulae from pressure and thermal dilution studies: clinical experience in forearm fistulae. *Clin Nephrol* 1985; 23:189-197 (evidence level: B)
20. Aldridge C, Greenwood RN, Cattell WR, Barrett RV. The assessment of arteriovenous fistulae created for haemodialysis from pressure and thermal dilution measurements. *J Med Eng Technol* 1984; 8:118-124 (evidence level: B)
21. Schwab SJ, Raymond JR, Saeed M, Newman GE, Dennis PA, Bollinger RR. Prevention of hemodialysis fistula thrombosis. Early detection of venous stenoses. *Kidney Int* 1989; 36:707-711 (evidence level: B)
22. Besarab A, Sullivan KL, Ross RP, Moritz MJ. Utility of intra-access pressure monitoring in detecting and correcting venous outlet stenoses prior to thrombosis. *Kidney Int* 1995; 47:1364-1373 (evidence level: B)
23. McCarley P, Wingard RL, Shyr Y, Pettus W, Hakim RM, Ikizler TA. Vascular access blood flow monitoring reduces access morbidity and costs. *Kidney Int* 2001; 60:1164-1172 (evidence level: B)
24. Kleinekofort W, Kraemer M, Rode C, Wizemann V. Extracorporeal pressure monitoring and the detection of vascular access stenosis. *Int J Artif Organs* 2002; 25:45-50
25. Besarab A, Frinak S, Sherman RA, Goldman J, Dumler F, Devita MV, Kapoian T, Al Saghir F, Lubkowski T. Simplified measurement of intra-access pressure. *J Am Soc Nephrol* 1998; 9:284-289 (evidence level: B)
26. Smits JH, van der Linden J, Hagen EC, Modderkolk-Cammeraat EC, Feith GW, Koomans HA, van den Dorpel MA, Blankestijn PJ. Graft surveillance: venous pressure, access flow, or the combination? *Kidney Int* 2001; 59:1551-1558 (evidence level: A)
27. Besarab A. Preventing vascular access dysfunction: which policy to follow. *Blood Purif* 2002; 20:26-35 (evidence level: C)
28. Hasbargen JA, Weaver DT, Hasbargen BJ. The effect of needle gauge on recirculation, venous pressure and bleeding from puncture sites. *Clin Nephrol* 1995; 44:322-324 (evidence level: A-B)
29. Shackleton CR, Taylor DC, Buckley AR, Rowley VA, Cooperberg PL, Fry PD. Predicting failure in polytetrafluoroethylene vascular access grafts for hemodialysis: a pilot study. *Can J Surg* 1987; 30:442-444 (evidence level: B)

30. Gadallah MF, Paulson WD, Vickers B, Work J. Accuracy of Doppler ultrasound in diagnosing anatomic stenosis of hemodialysis arteriovenous access as compared with fistulography. *Am J Kidney Dis* 1998; 32:273-277 (evidence level: A)
31. MacDonald MJ, Martin LG, Hughes JD, Kikeri D, Scout DC, Harker LA Distribution and severity of stenoses in functioning arterioivenous grafts: a duplex and angiographic study. *J Vasc Technol* 1996; 20:131-136
32. Wittenberg G, Schindler T, Tschammler A, Kenn W, Hahn D. [Value of color-coded duplex ultrasound in evaluating arm blood vessels-arteries and hemodialysis shunts]. *Ultraschall Med 1998; 19:22-27 (evidence level: B)*
33. Bacchini G, Cappello A, La Milia V, Andrulli S, Locatelli F. Color doppler ultrasonography imaging to guide transluminal angioplasty of venous stenosis. *Kidney Int* 2000; 58:1810-1813 (evidence level: B)
34. Hartnell GG, Hughes LA, Finn JP, Longmaid HE, III. Magnetic resonance angiography of the central chest veins. A new gold standard? *Chest* 1995; 107:1053-1057 (evidence level: B)
35. Kroencke TJ, Taupitz M, Arnold R, Fritsche L, Hamm B. Three-dimensional gadolinium-enhanced magnetic resonance venography in suspected thrombo-occlusive disease of the central chest veins. *Chest* 2001; 120:1570-1576 (evidence level: B)

References – Management of A/V Fistula Stenosis

1. Turmel-Rodrigues L, Pengloan J, Baudin S, Testou D, Abaza M, Dahdah G, Mouton A, Blanchard D. Treatment of stenosis and thrombosis in haemodialysis fistulas and grafts by interventional radiology. *Nephrol Dial Transplant* 2000; 15:2029-2036 (evidence level: B)
2. Turmel-Rodrigues L, Pengloan J, Blanchier D, Abaza M, Birmele B, Haillot O, Blanchard D. Insufficient dialysis shunts: improved long-term patency rates with close hemodynamic monitoring, repeated percutaneous balloon angioplasty, and stent placement. *Radiology* 1993; 187:273-278 (evidence level: B)
3. Langeveld APM, Leunissen KML, Eikelboom BC, Kitslaar PJEHM. Duplex ultrasound detection of stenoses in newly created hemodialysis A/V fistulas. Maastricht 1990; 145-154 (evidence level: B)
4. Turmel-Rodrigues L, Raynaud A, Bourquelot P. Percutaneous treatment of arteriovenous access dysfunction. in: Hemodialysis Vascular Access: Practice and Problems. Conlon PJ, Schwab SJ, Nicholson ML (eds). Oxford, New York Oxford University Press 2000; 183-202
5. Schwab SJ, Raymond JR, Saeed M, Newman GE, Dennis PA, Bollinger RR. Prevention of hemodialysis fistula thrombosis. Early detection of venous stenoses. *Kidney Int* 1989; 36:707-711 (evidence level: B)
6. Romero A, Polo JR, Garcia ME, Garcia Sabrido JL, Quintans A, Ferreiroa JP. Salvage of angioaccess after late thrombosis of radiocephalic fistulas for hemodialysis. *Int Surg* 1986; 71:122-124 (evidence level: B)
7. Clark TW, Hirsch DA, Jindal KJ, Veugelers PJ, LeBlanc J. Outcome and prognostic factors of restenosis after percutaneous treatment of native hemodialysis fistulas. *J Vasc Interv Radiol* 2002; 13:51-59

8. Vorwerk D, Adam G, Muller-Leisse C, Guenther RW. Hemodialysis fistulas and grafts: use of cutting balloons to dilate venous stenoses. *Radiology* 1996; 201:864-867 (evidence level: B)

References – Management of A/V Fistula Thrombosis

1. Romero A, Polo JR, Garcia ME, Garcia Sabrido JL, Quintans A, Ferreiroa JP. Salvage of angioaccess after late thrombosis of radiocephalic fistulas for hemodialysis. *Int Surg* 1986; 71:122-124 (evidence level: B)
2. Oakes DD, Sherck JP, Cobb LF. Surgical salvage of failed radiocephalic arteriovenous fistulae: techniques and results in 29 patients. *Kidney Int* 1998; 53:480-487 (evidence level: B)
3. Turmel-Rodrigues L, Pengloan J, Rodrigue H, Brillet G, Lataste A, Pierre D, Jourdan JL, Blanchard D. Treatment of failed native arteriovenous fistulae for hemodialysis by interventional radiology. *Kidney Int* 2000; 57:1124-1140 (evidence level: B)
4. Turmel-Rodrigues L, Sapoval M, Pengloan J, Billaux L, Testou D, Hauss S, Mouton A, Blanchard D. Manual thromboaspiration and dilation of thrombosed dialysis access: mid-term results of a simple concept. *J Vasc Interv Radiol* 1997; 8: 813-824
5. Haage P, Vorwerk D, Wildberger JE, Piroth W, Schurmann K, Gunther RW.. Percutaneous treatment of thrombosed primary arteriovenous hemodialysis access fistulae. *Kidney Int* 2000; 57: 1169-1175
6. Schon D, Mishler R. Salvage of occluded autologous arteriovenous fistulae. *Am J Kidney Dis* 2000; 36: 804-810
7. Schmitz-Rode T, Wildberger JE, Hubner D, Wein B, Schurmann K, Gunther RW. Recanalization of thrombosed dialysis access with use of a rotating mini-pigtail catheter: follow-up study. *J Vasc Interv Radiol* 2000; 11: 721-727
8. Rocek M, Peregrin JH, Lasovickova J, Krajickova D, Slaviokova M. Mechanical thrombolysis of thrombosed hemodialysis native fistulas with use of the Arrow-Trerotola percutaneous thrombolytic device: our preliminary experience. *J Vasc Interv Radiol* 2000; 11: 1153-1158
9. Zaleski GX, Funaki B, Kenney S, Lorenz JM, Garofalo R. Angioplasty and bolus urokinase infusion for the restoration of function in thrombosed Brescia-Cimino dialysis fistulas. *J Vasc Interv Radiol* 1999; 10: 129-136
10. Rousseau H, Sapoval M, Ballini P et al. Percutaneous recanalization of acutely thrombosed vessels by hydrodynamic thrombectomy (Hydrolyser). *Eur.Radiol.* 1997; 7: 935-941
11. Overbosch EH, Pattynama PM, Aarts HJ et al. Occluded hemodialysis shunts: Dutch multicenter experience with the hydrolyser catheter. *Radiology* 1996; 201: 485-488
12. Liang HL, Pan HB, Chung HM et al. Restoration of thrombosed Brescia-Cimino dialysis fistulas by using percutaneous transluminal angioplasty. *Radiology* 2002; 223: 339-344
13. Manninen HI, Kaukanen ET, Ikaheimo R et al. Brachial arterial access: endovascular treatment of failing Brescia-Cimino hemodialysis fistulas--initial success and long-term results. *Radiology* 2001; 218: 711-718
14. Turmel-Rodrigues L., Raynaud A., Bourquelot P. Percutaneous treatment of arteriovenous access dysfunction. In: Conlon P.J., Schwab S.J., Nicholson M.L., eds. He-

modialysis Vascular Access: Practice and Problems. Oxford University Press, Oxford, New York: 2000: 183-202 (evidence level: C)

References – Management of A/V Fistula Infection after 1st Month of Placement

1. Canaud B., Kessler M., Pedrini MT, Tattersall JE, ter Wee P.M., Vanholder R, Wanner C. European Best Practice Guidelines - Dialysis. *Nephrol Dial Transplant* 2002. Suppl. 7
2. McCarthy JT and Steckelberg JM. Infective endocarditis in patients receiving long-term hemodialysis. *Mayo Clin Proc* 2000; 75:1008-1014 (evidence level: B)
3. Kovalik EC, Raymond JR, Albers FJ, Berkoben M, Butterly DW, Montella B, Conlon PJ. A clustering of epidural abscesses in chronic hemodialysis patients: risks of salvaging access catheters in cases of infection. *J Am Soc Nephrol* 1996; 7:2264-2267 (evidence level: B)
4. Obrador GT and Levenson DJ. Spinal epidural abscess in hemodialysis patients: report of three cases and review of the literature. *Am J Kidney Dis* 1996; 27:75-83 (evidence level: B)
5. Tordoir JH, Kwan TS, Herman JM, Carol EJ, Jakimowicz JJ. Primary and secondary access surgery for haemodialysis with the Brescia- Cimino fistula and the polytetrafluoroethylene (PTFE) graft. *Neth J Surg* 1983; 35:8-12 (evidence level: B)
6. Fong IW, Capellan JM, Simbul M, Angel J. Infection of arterio-venous fistulas created for chronic haemodialysis. *Scand J Infect Dis* 1993; 25:215-220 (evidence level : B)
7. Nassar GM and Ayus JC. Infectious complications of the hemodialysis access. *Kidney Int* 2001; 60:1-13 (evidence level: C)

References – Management of Graft Stenosis

1. Jindal KK, Ethier JH, Lindsay RM, Barre PE, Kappel JE, Carlisle EJ, Common A. Clinical practice guidelines for vascular access. Canadian Society of Nephrology. *J Am Soc Nephrol* 1999; 10 Suppl 13:S297-S305 (evidence level: C)
2. Depner TA. Techniques for prospective detection of venous stenosis. *Adv Ren Replace Ther* 1994; 1:119-130 (evidence level: C)
3. Beathard GA. Percutaneous transvenous angioplasty in the treatment of vascular access stenosis. *Kidney Int* 1992; 42:1390-1397 (evidence level: B)
4. Puckett JW and Lindsay SF. Midgraft curettage as a routine adjunct to salvage operations for thrombosed polytetrafluoroethylene hemodialysis access grafts. *Am J Surg* 1988; 156:139-143 (evidence level: B)
5. Dickermann R, Robison J, Seigel J. Incidence and causes of access failure. ChicagoPrecept Press 1995; 3-15
6. Dougherty MJ, Calligaro KD, Schindler N, Raviola CA, Ntoso A. Endovascular versus surgical treatment for thrombosed hemodialysis grafts: A prospective, randomized study. *J Vasc Surg* 1999; 30:1016-1023 (evidence level: A)
7. Marston WA, Criado E, Jaques PF, Mauro MA, Burnham SJ, Keagy BA. Prospective randomized comparison of surgical versus endovascular management of thrombosed dialysis access grafts. *J Vasc Surg* 1997; 26:373-380 (evidence level: A)

8. Vega MD, Polo M, Jr., Flores A, Rueda JA, Lopez Baena JA, Garcia PR, Gonzalez TE. [Proximal vein by-pass in the treatment of venous stenosis in expanded polytetrafluoroethylene prosthesis for hemodialysis]. *Rev Clin Esp* 2000; 200:64-68 (evidence level: B)
9. Polo JR, Polo J, Vega D, Pacccheco D, Gracia-Pajares R. Surgical treatment of stenosis and thrombosis in dialysis grafts. *Dialyse-Journal* 1999; 66:242-245 (evidence level:C)
10. Vorwerk D, Guenther RW, Mann H, Bohndorf K, Keulers P, Alzen G, Sohn M, Kistler D. Venous stenosis and occlusion in hemodialysis shunts: follow-up results of stent placement in 65 patients. *Radiology* 1995; 195:140-146 (evidence level: B)
11. Turmel-Rodrigues L, Pengloan J, Blanchier D, Abaza M, Birmele B, Haillot O, Blanchard D. Insufficient dialysis shunts: improved long-term patency rates with close hemodynamic monitoring, repeated percutaneous balloon angioplasty, and stent placement. *Radiology* 1993; 187:273-278 (evidence level: B)
12. Murray BM, Rajczak S, Ali B, Herman A, Mepani B. Assessment of access blood flow after preemptive angioplasty. *Am J Kidney Dis* 2001; 37:1029-1038 (evidence level: B)
13. Ahya SN, Windus DW, Vesely TM. Flow in hemodialysis grafts after angioplasty: Do radiologic criteria predict success? *Kidney Int* 2001; 59:1974-1978 (evidence level: B)
14. an der Linden J, Smits JH, Assink JH, Wolterbeek DW, Zijlstra JJ, de Jong GH, van den Dorpel MA, Blankestijn PJ. Short- and long-term functional effects of percutaneous transluminal angioplasty in hemodialysis vascular access. *J Am Soc Nephrol* 2002; 13:715-720 (evidence level: B)

References – Management of Graft Thrombosis

1. Dougherty MJ, Calligaro KD, Schindler N, Raviola CA, Ntoso A. Endovascular versus surgical treatment for thrombosed hemodialysis grafts: A prospective, randomized study. *J Vasc Surg* 1999; 30:1016-1023 (evidence level: A)
2. Marston WA, Criado E, Jaques PF, Mauro MA, Burnham SJ, Keagy BA. Prospective randomized comparison of surgical versus endovascular management of thrombosed dialysis access grafts. *J Vasc Surg* 1997; 26:373-380 (evidence level: A)
3. Farner MC. Regarding "Endovascular versus surgical treatment for thrombosed hemodialysis: a prospective, randomized study". *J Vasc.Surg.* 2000; 32: 1038-1039
4. Turmel-Rodrigues L, Vesely T, Bourquelot P, Cooper S, Konner K, Pengloan J, Raynaud A, Sapoval M, Sofocleous C, Tordoir J, Trerotola S, Vorwerk D . Regarding "Prospective randomized comparison of surgical versus endovascular management of thrombosed dialysis access grafts". *J Vasc.Surg.* 1998; 28: 384-386
5. Turmel-Rodrigues L, Pengloan J, Baudin S, Testou D, Abaza M, Dahdah G, Mouton A, Blanchard D. Treatment of stenosis and thrombosis in haemodialysis fistulas and grafts by interventional radiology. *Nephrol Dial Transplant* 2000; 15:2029-2036 (evidence level: B)
6. III. NKF-K/DOQI Clinical Practice Guidelines for Vascular Access: update 2000. *Am J Kidney Dis* 2001; 37 (Suppl. 1) : S137-S181
7. Hodges TC, Fillinger MF, Zwolak RM, Walsh DB, Bech F, Cronenwett JL. Longitudinal comparison of dialysis access methods: risk factors for failure. *J Vasc Surg* 1997; 26:1009-1019

8. Vesely TM, Williams D, Weiss M, Hicks M, Stainken B, Matalon T, Dolmatch B. Comparison of the angiojet rheolytic catheter to surgical thrombectomy for the treatment of thrombosed hemodialysis grafts. Peripheral AngioJet Clinical Trial. *J Vasc Interv Radiol* 1999; 10:1195-1205
9. Smits HF, Smits JH, Wust AF, Buskens E, Blankestijn PJ. Percutaneous thrombolysis of thrombosed haemodialysis access grafts: comparison of three mechanical devices. *Nephrol Dial Transplant* 2002; 17:467-473 (evidence level: B)
10. Beathard GA. Mechanical versus pharmacomechanical thrombolysis for the treatment of thrombosed dialysis access grafts. *Kidney Int* 1994; 45:1401-1406 (evidence level: A-B)
11. Albertov, Mansilla, Toombs BD, Vaughn WK, Zeledon JI. Patency and life-spans of failing hemodialysis grafts in patients undergoing repeated percutaneous de-clotting. *Tex Heart Inst J* 2001; 28:249-253 (evidence level: B)
12. Turmel-Rodrigues L, Raynaud A, Bourquelot P. Percutaneous treatment of arteriovenous access dysfunction. in: Hemodialysis Vascular Access: Practice and Problems. Conlon PJ, Schwab SJ, Nicholson ML (eds). Oxford, New York Oxford University Press 2000; 183-202 (evidence level: C)

References – Management of Graft Infection after 1st Month of Placement (1)

1. Nassar GM and Ayus JC. Clotted arteriovenous grafts: a silent source of infection. *Semin Dial* 2000; 13:1-3 (evidence level: C)
2. Nassar GM and Ayus JC. Infectious complications of the hemodialysis access. *Kidney Int* 2001; 60:1-13 (evidence level: C)
3. Kessler M, Canaud B, Pedrini MT, Tattersall JE, ter Wee P.M, Vanholder R, Wanner C. European Best Practice Guidelines - Dialysis. *Nephrol Dial Transplant* 2002; (evidence level: C)
4. Taylor B, Sigley RD, May KJ. Fate of infected and eroded hemodialysis grafts and autogenous fistulas. *Am J Surg* 1993; 165:632-636 (evidence level: B)
5. Schwab DP, Taylor SM, Cull DL, Langan EM, III, Snyder BA, Sullivan TM, Youkey JR. Isolated arteriovenous dialysis access graft segment infection: the results of segmental bypass and partial graft excision. *Ann Vasc Surg* 2000; 14:63-66 (evidence level: B)
6. Padberg FT, Jr., Lee BC, Curl GR. Hemoaccess site infection. *Surg Gynecol Obstet* 1992; 174:103-108 (evidence level: B)

References – Management of Graft Infection after 1st Month of Placement (2)

1. Obrador GT and Levenson DJ. Spinal epidural abscess in hemodialysis patients: report of three cases and review of the literature. *Am J Kidney Dis* 1996; 27:75-83 (evidence level: B)
2. Kovalik EC, Raymond JR, Albers FJ, Berkoben M, Butterly DW, Montella B, Conlon PJ. A clustering of epidural abscesses in chronic hemodialysis patients: risks of salvaging access catheters in cases of infection. *J Am Soc Nephrol* 1996; 7:2264-2267 (evidence level: B)
3. Minga TE, Flanagan KH, Allon M. Clinical consequences of infected arteriovenous grafts in hemodialysis patients. *Am J Kidney Dis* 2001; 38:975-978 (evidence level: B)

4. Mohamed M, Habte-Gabr E, Mueller W. Infected arteriovenous hemodialysis graft presenting as left and right infective endocarditis. *Am J Nephrol* 1995; 15:521-523 (evidence level: B)
5. Besarab A. Preventing vascular access dysfunction: which policy to follow. *Blood Purif* 2002; 20:26-35 (evidence level: C)
6. Nassar GM and Ayus JC. Infectious complications of the hemodialysis access. Kidney Int 2001; 60:1-13 (evidence level: C)
7. Matsuura JH, Johansen KH, Rosenthal D, Clark MD, Clarke KA, Kirby LB. Cryopreserved femoral vein grafts for difficult hemodialysis access. *Ann Vasc Surg* 2000; 14:50-55 (evidence level: B)
8. Deneuville M. Infection of PTFE grafts used to create arteriovenous fistulas for hemodialysis access. *Ann Vasc Surg* 2000; 14:473-479 (evidence level: B)

References – Management of Aneurysms

1. Henry M.L. Options for restoring of thrombosed vascular access: surgery. in: Hemodialysis Vascular Access: Practice and Problems. Conlon PJ, Schwab SJ, Nicholson ML (eds). Oxford, New York Oxford University Press 2000; 227-239
2. III. NKF-K/DOQI Clinical Practice Guidelines for Vascular Access: update 2000. *Am J Kidney Dis* 2001; 37:S137-S181

References – Management of High Flow in A/V Fistula and Graft

1. Turmel-Rodrigues L, Raynaud A, Bourquelot P. Percutaneous treatment of arteriovenous access dysfunction. in: Hemodialysis Vascular Access: Practice and Problems. Conlon PJ, Schwab SJ, Nicholson ML (eds). Oxford, New York Oxford University Press 2000; 183-202 (evidence level: C)
2. Dikow R, Schwenger V, Zeier M, Ritz E. Do AV Fistulas Contribute to Cardiac Mortaltity in Hemodialysis Patients? *Semin Dial* 2002; 15:14-17 (evidence level: C)
3. Murphy GJ, White SA, Knight AJ, Doughman T, Nicholson ML. Long-term results of arteriovenous fistulas using transposed autologous basilic vein. *Br J Surg* 2000; 87:819-823 (evidence level: B)
4. Ono K, Muto Y, Yano K, Yukizane T. Anterior chest wall axillary artery to contralateral axillary vein graft for vascular access in hemodialysis. *Artif Organs* 1995; 19:1233-1236 (evidence level: B)
5. Engelberts I, Tordoir JH, Boorgu R, Schreij G. High-Output Cardiac Failure due to Excessive Shunting in a Hemodialysis Access Fistula: An Easily Overlooked Diagnosis. *Am J Nephrol* 1995; 15:323-326 (evidence level: B)
6. Munclinger M, Nemecek K, Serf B, Vondracek V, Hrudova J. Effect of arteriovenous fistula creation and maturation on rest hemodynamics in patients with end-stage renal disease. *Nephron* 1987; 46:105-106 (evidence level: B)
7. Pandeya S, Lindsay RM. The relationship between cardiac output and access flow during hemodialysis. *ASAIO J* 1999; 45: 135-138
8. Young PR, Jr., Rohr MS, Marterre WF, Jr. High-output cardiac failure secondary to a brachiocephalic arteriovenous hemodialysis fistula: two cases. *Am Surg* 1998; 64:239-241 (evidence level: B)
9. Bourquelot P, Corbi P, Cussenot O. Surgical improvement of high flow fistulas. Pluribus Press (USA). Edited by Sommer B, Henry M.L: 1989; 124-130

10. Bourquelot P. High flow - surgical treatment. *Blood Purif* 2001; 19:130-131 (evidence level: C)

References – Management of Ischaemia (1)

1. Levine M.P. The hemodialysis patient and hand amputation. *Am J Nephrol* 2001; 21:498-501 (evidence level: B)
2. Lin G, Kais H, Halpern Z, Chayen D, Weissgarten J, Negri M, Cohn M, Averbukh J, Halevy A. Pulse oxymetry evaluation of oxygen saturation in the upper extremity with an arteriovenous fistula before and during hemodialysis. *Am J Kidney Dis* 1997; 29:230-232 (evidence level: B)
3. Odland MD, Kelly PH, Ney AL, Andersen RC, Bubrick MP. Management of dialysis-associated steal syndrome complicating upper extremity arteriovenous fistulas: use of intraoperative digital photoplethysmography. *Surgery* 1991; 110:664-669 (evidence level: B)
4. Hye RJ and Wolf YG. Ischemic monomelic neuropathy: an under-recognized complication of hemodialysis access. *Ann Vasc Surg* 1994; 8:578-582 (evidence level: B)
5. Valji K, Hye RJ, Roberts AC, Oglevie SB, Ziegler T, Bookstein JJ. Hand ischemia in patients with hemodialysis access grafts: angiographic diagnosis and treatment. *Radiology* 1995; 196:697-701 (evidence level: B)
6. Miles AM. Upper limb ischemia after vascular access surgery: differential diagnosis and management. *Semin Dial* 2000; 13:312-315 (evidence level: C)
7. DeCaprio JD, Valentine RJ, Kakish HB, Awad R, Hagino RT, Clagett GP. Steal syndrome complicating hemodialysis access. *Cardiovasc Surg* 1997; 5:648-653 (evidence level: B)
8. Halevy A, Halpern Z, Negri M, Hod G, Weissgarten J, Averbukh Z, Modai D. Pulse oximetry in the evaluation of the painful hand after arteriovenous fistula creation. *J Vasc Surg* 1991; 14:537-539 (evidence level: B)
9. Raynaud A. Distal ischemia: radiological approach. *Dialyse-Journal* 1999; 66:261-263 (evidence level: C)
10. Guerra A, Raynaud A, Beyssen B, Pagny JY, Sapoval M, Angel C. Arterial percutaneous angioplasty in upper limbs with vascular access devices for haemodialysis. *Nephrol Dial Transplant* 2002; 17:843-851 (evidence level B)

References – Management of Ischaemia (2)

1. Haimov M, Schanzer H, Skladani M. Pathogenesis and management of upper-extremity ischemia following angioaccess surgery. *Blood Purif* 1996; 14:350-354 (evidence level: B)
2. DeCaprio JD, Valentine RJ, Kakish HB, Awad R, Hagino RT, Clagett GP. Steal syndrome complicating hemodialysis access. *Cardiovasc Surg* 1997; 5:648-653 (evidence level: B)
3. Odland MD, Kelly PH, Ney AL, Andersen RC, Bubrick MP. Management of dialysis-associated steal syndrome complicating upper extremity arteriovenous fistulas: use of intraoperative digital photoplethysmography. *Surgery* 1991; 110:664-669 (evidence level: B)

4. Rivers SP, Scher LA, Veith FJ. Correction of steal syndrome secondary to hemodialysis access fistulas: a simplified quantitative technique. *Surgery* 1992; 112:593-597 (evidence level: B)
5. Bussell JA, Abbott JA, Lim RC. A radial steal syndrome with arteriovenous fistula for hemodialysis. Studies in seven patients. *Ann Intern Med* 1971; 75:387-394 (evidence level: B)
6. Chemla E, Raynaud A, Carreres T, Sapoval M, Beyssen B, Bourquelot P, Gaux JC. Preoperative assessment of the efficacy of distal radial artery ligation in treatment of steal syndrome complicating access for hemodialysis. *Ann Vasc Surg* 1999; 13:618-621
7. Berman SS, Gentile AT, Glickman MH, Mills JL, Hurwitz RL, Westerband A, Marek JM, Hunter GC, McEnroe CS, Fogle MA, Stokes GK. Distal revascularization-interval ligation for limb salvage and maintenance of dialysis access in ischemic steal syndrome. *J Vasc Surg* 1997; 26:393-402 (evidence level: B)

References – Management of Central Venous Obstruction (1)

1. Sottiurai VS, Stephens A, Champagne L, Reisen E. Preservation of hemodialysis access with central obstruction. *Int J Angiol* 1996; 5:171-174 (evidence level: B)
2. Bhatia DS, Money SR, Ochsner JL, Crockett DE, Chatman D, Dharamsey SA, Mulingtapang RF, Shaw D, Ramee SR. Comparison of surgical bypass and percutaneous balloon dilatation with primary stent placement in the treatment of central venous obstruction in the dialysis patient: one-year follow-up. *Ann Vasc Surg* 1996; 10:452-455 (evidence level: B)
3. Landwehr P, Tschammler A, Schaefer RM, Lackner K. [The value of color-coded duplex sonography of a dialysis shunt]. *Rofo Fortschr Geb Rontgenstr Neuen Bildgeb Verfahr* 1990; 153:185-191 (evidence level: A)
4. Dousset V, Grenier N, Douws C, Senuita P, Sassouste G, Ada L, Potaux L. Hemodialysis grafts: color Doppler flow imaging correlated with digital subtraction angiography and functional status. *Radiology* 1991; 181:89-94 (evidence level: B)
5. Losinno F, Busato F, Degli EE, Pavlica P, Spongano M, Viglietta G. [Angiographic study of the complications of vascular access in patients under hemodialysis]. *Radiol Med (Torino)* 1988; 75:621-625 (evidence level: B)
6. MacDonald MJ, Martin LG, Hughes JD, Kikeri D, Scout DC, Harker LA. Distribution and severity of stenoses in functioning arterioivenous grafts: a duplex and angiographic study. *J Vasc Technol* 1996; 20:131-136
7. Ortega O, Rodriguez I, Gallar P, Gimenez E, Oliet A, Vigil A. A simple method for structural assessment of hemodialysis fistulas. 10-year experience. *Nephrologia* 1999; 19:428-433 (evidence level: B)
8. Elduayen B, Martinez-Cuesta A, Vivas I., Alonso C., Velazquez P., Ignacio B.J. Venous stenoses on patients undergoing hemodialysis. Treatment by self-expanding metallic stents. *Radiologia* 1999; 41:351-355 (evidence level: B)
9. Pedrini L, Pisano E, Sensi L, Isceri S. Superior vena cava thrombosis secondary to thoracic outlet syndrome. Case report. Int Angiol 2000; 19:366-368 (evidence level: B)
10. Urschel HC, Jr. and Razzuk MA. Paget-Schroetter syndrome: what is the best management? *Ann Thorac Surg* 2000; 69:1663-1668 (evidence level: A)
11. Money S, Bhatia D, Daharamsay S, Mulingtapan R, Shaw D, Ramee S. Comparison of surgical by-pass, percutaneous balloon dilatation (PTA) and PTA with stent

placement in the treatment of venous occlusion in the dialysis patient. One year follow up (abstract). *Int Angiol* 1995; 14:176 (evidence level: B)
12. Quinn SF, Schuman ES, Demlow TA, Standage BA, Ragsdale JW, Green GS, Sheley RC. Percutaneous transluminal angioplasty versus endovascular stent placement in the treatment of venous stenoses in patients undergoing hemodialysis: intermediate results. *J Vasc Interv Radiol* 1995; 6:851-855 (evidence level: A-B)
13. Haage P, Vorwerk D, Piroth W, Schuermann K, Guenther RW. Treatment of hemodialysis-related central venous stenosis or occlusion: results of primary Wallstent placement and follow-up in 50 patients. *Radiology* 1999; 212:175-180 (evidence level: B)
14. Mickley V. [Stent or bypass? Treatment results in benign central venous obstruction]. *Zentralbl Chir* 2001; 126:445-449 (evidence level: B)
15. Turmel-Rodrigues L, Raynaud A, Bourquelot P. Percutaneous treatment of arteriovenous access dysfunction. in: Hemodialysis Vascular Access: Practice and Problems. Conlon PJ, Schwab SJ, Nicholson ML (eds). Oxford, New York Oxford University Press 2000; 183-202 (evidence level: C)
16. Turmel-Rodrigues L, Pengloan J, Bourquelot P. Interventional radiology in hemodialysis fistulae and grafts: a multidisciplinary approach. *Cardiovasc Intervent Radiol* 2002; 25:3-16
17. Schindler J, Bona RD, Chen HH, Feingold JM, Edwards RL, Tutschka PJ, Bilgrami S. Regional thrombolysis with urokinase for central venous catheter- related thrombosis in patients undergoing high-dose chemotherapy with autologous blood stem cell rescue. *Clin Appl Thromb Hemost* 1999; 5:25-29 (evidence level: B)
18. dwards RD and Jackson JE. Case report: superior vena caval obstruction treated by thrombolysis, mechanical thrombectomy and metallic stents. *Clin Radiol* 1993; 48:215-217 (evidence level: B)
19. Fraschini G, Jadeja J, Lawson M, Holmes FA, Carrasco HC, Wallace S. Local infusion of urokinase for the lysis of thrombosis associated with permanent central venous catheters in cancer patients. *J Clin Oncol* 1987; 5:672-678 (evidence level: B)

References – Management of Central Venous Obstruction (2)

1. Mickley V. [Stent or bypass? Treatment results in benign central venous obstruction]. *Zentralbl Chir* 2001; 126:445-449 (evidence level: B)
2. Sottiurai VS, Stephens A, Champagne L, Reisen E. Preservation of hemodialysis access with central obstruction. *Int J Angiol* 1996; 5:171-174 (evidence level: B)
3. Ono K, Muto Y, Yano K, Yukizane T. Anterior chest wall axillary artery to contralateral axillary vein graft for vascular access in hemodialysis. *Artif Organs* 1995; 19:1233-1236 (evidence level: B)
4. Dracon M, Watine O, Pruvot F, Noel C, Lelievre G. [Axillo-axillary access in hemodialysis]. *Nephrologie* 1994; 15:175-176 (evidence level: B)
5. Polo JR, Sanabia J, Garcia-Sabrido JL, Luno J, Menarguez C, Echenagusia A. Brachial-jugular polytetrafluoroethylene fistulas for hemodialysis. *Am J Kidney Dis* 1990; 16:465-468 (evidence level: B)
6. Myers JL and Mukherjee D. Bypass graft to the contralateral internal jugular vein for venous outflow obstruction of a functioning hemodialysis access fistula. *J Vasc Surg* 2000; 32:818-820 (evidence level: B)

7. Korzets A, Ori Y, Baytner S, Zevin D, Chagnac A, Weinstein T, Herman M, Agmon M, Gafter U. The femoral artery-femoral vein polytetrafluoroethylene graft: a 14-year retrospective study. *Nephrol Dial Transplant* 1998; 13:1215-1220 (evidence level: B)
8. Duncan JM, Baldwin RT, Caralis JP, Cooley DA. Subclavian vein-to-right atrial bypass for symptomatic venous hypertension. *Ann Thorac Surg* 1991; 52:1342-1343 (evidence level: B)
9. El Sabrout RA and Duncan JM. Right atrial bypass grafting for central venous obstruction associated with dialysis access: another treatment option. *J Vasc Surg* 1999; 29:472-478 (evidence level: B)
10. Mickley V. Subclavian artery to right atrium haemodialysis bridge graft for superior vena caval occlusion. *Nephrol Dial Transplant* 1996; 11:1361-1362 (evidence level: B)
11. Criado E, Marston WA, Jaques PF, Mauro MA, Keagy BA. Proximal venous outflow obstruction in patients with upper extremity arteriovenous dialysis access. *Ann Vasc Surg* 1994; 8:530-535 (evidence level: B)

References – Identification and Management of Tunneled Catheter Complications

1. Schwab SJ and Beathard G. The hemodialysis catheter conundrum: hate living with them, but can't live without them. *Kidney Int* 1999; 56:1-17 (evidence level: C)
2. Depner TA, Rizwan S, Stasi TA. Pressure effects on roller pump blood flow during hemodialysis. *ASAIO Trans* 1990; 36:M456-M459 (evidence level: B)
3. O'Riordan E and Conlon PJ. Haemodialysis catheter bacteraemia: evolving strategies. *Curr Opin Nephrol Hypertens* 1998; 7:639-642 (evidence level: C)
4. Kite P, Dobbins BM, Wilcox MH, Fawley WN, Kindon AJ, Thomas D, Tighe MJ, McMahon MJ. Evaluation of a novel endoluminal brush method for in situ diagnosis of catheter related sepsis. *J Clin Pathol* 1997; 50:278-282 (evidence level: B)
5. Rotellar C, Sims SC, Freeland J, Korba J, Jessen M, Taylor A. Right atrium thrombosis in patients on hemodialysis. *Am J Kidney Dis* 1996; 27:726-728 (evidence level: B)
6. Seddon PA, Hrinya MK, Gaynord MA, Lion CM, Mangold BM, Bruns FJ. Effectiveness of low dose urokinase on dialysis catheter thrombolysis. *ASAIO J* 1998; 44:M559-M561 (evidence level: B)
7. Clase CM, Crowther MA, Ingram AJ, Cina CS. Thrombolysis for restoration of patency to haemodialysis central venous catheters: a systematic review. *J Thromb Thrombolysis* 2001; 11:127-136 (evidence level: C)
8. Twardowski ZJ. High-dose intradialytic urokinase to restore the patency of permanent central vein hemodialysis catheters. *Am J Kidney Dis* 1998; 31:841-847 (evidence level: B)
9. Northsea C. Continuous quality improvement: improving hemodialysis catheter patency using urokinase. *ANNA J* 1996; 23:567-71, 615 (evidence level: C)
10. Suhocki PV, Conlon PJ, Jr., Knelson MH, Harland R, Schwab SJ. Silastic cuffed catheters for hemodialysis vascular access: thrombolytic and mechanical correction of malfunction. *Am J Kidney Dis* 1996; 28:379-386 (evidence level: B)
11. Hannah A and Buttimore AL. Thrombolysis of blocked hemodialysis catheter using recombinant tissue-type plasminogen activator. *Nephron* 1991; 59:517-518 (evidence level: B)

12. Paulsen D, Reisoether A, Aasen M, Fauchald P. Use of tissue plasminogen activator for reopening of clotted dialysis catheters. *Nephron* 1993; 64:468-470 (evidence level: B)
13. Daeihagh P, Jordan J, Chen J, Rocco M. Efficacy of tissue plasminogen activator administration on patency of hemodialysis access catheters. *Am J Kidney Dis* 2000; 36:75-79 (evidence level: B)
14. Falk A, Mitty H, Guller J, Teodorescu V, Uribarri J, Vassalotti J. Thrombolysis of clotted hemodialysis grafts with tissue-type plasminogen activator. *J Vasc Interv Radiol* 2001; 12:305-311 (evidence level: B)
15. Ponec D, Irwin D, Haire WD, Hill PA, Li X, McCluskey ER. Recombinant tissue plasminogen activator (alteplase) for restoration of flow in occluded central venous access devices: a double-blind placebo-controlled trial-the Cardiovascular Thrombolytic to Open Occluded Lines (COOL) efficacy trial. *J Vasc Interv Radiol* 2001; 12:951-955 (evidence level: A)
16. Savader SJ, Haikal LC, Ehrman KO, Porter DJ, Oteham AC. Hemodialysis catheter-associated fibrin sheaths: treatment with a low - dose rt-PA infusion. *J Vasc Interv Radiol* 2000; 11:1131-1136 (evidence level: B)
17. Schenk P, Rosenkranz AR, Wolfl G, Horl WH, Traindl O. Recombinant tissue plasminogen activator is a useful alternative to heparin in priming quinton permcath. *Am J Kidney Dis* 2000; 35:130-136 (evidence level: B)
18. Little MA and Walshe JJ. A longitudinal study of the repeated use of alteplase as therapy for tunneled hemodialysis catheter dysfunction. *Am J Kidney Dis* 2002; 39:86-91 (evidence level: B)
19. Rockall AG, Harris A, Wetton CW, Taube D, Gedroyc W, Al Kutoubi MA. Stripping of failing haemodialysis catheters using the Amplatz gooseneck snare. *Clin Radiol* 1997; 52:616-620 (evidence level: B)
20. Crain MR, Mewissen MW, Ostrowski GJ, Paz-Fumagalli R, Beres RA, Wertz RA. Fibrin sleeve stripping for salvage of failing hemodialysis catheters: technique and initial results. *Radiology* 1996; 198:41-44 (evidence level: B)
21. Haskal ZJ, Leen VH, Thomas-Hawkins C, Shlansky-Goldberg RD, Baum RA, Soulen MC. Transvenous removal of fibrin sheaths from tunneled hemodialysis catheters. *J Vasc Interv Radiol* 1996; 7:513-517 (evidence level: B)
22. Gray RJ, Levitin A, Buck D, Brown LC, Sparling YH, Jablonski KA, Fessahaye A, Gupta AK. Percutaneous fibrin sheath stripping versus transcatheter urokinase infusion for malfunctioning well-positioned tunneled central venous dialysis catheters: a prospective, randomized trial. *J Vasc Interv Radiol* 2000; 11:1121-1129 (evidence level: A-B)
23. Garofalo RS, Zaleski GX, Lorenz JM, Funaki B, Rosenblum JD, Leef JA. Exchange of poorly functioning tunneled permanent hemodialysis catheters. *Am J Roentgenol* 1999; 173:155-158 (evidence level: B)
24. Kress L and Donoghue J. Catheter brushing has made a sweeping difference to our clinical practice. *Nephrol Nurs J* 2000; 27:403-405 (evidence level: B)
25. Bel'eed K, Kumar A, Asin M, Sellars L. Endoluminal brushing of blocked indwelling haemodialysis catheters. *Nephrol Dial Transplant* 1999; 14:241 (evidence level: B)
26. Tranter SA and Donoghue J. Brushing has made a sweeping change: use of the endoluminal FAS brush in haemodialysis central venous catheter management. *Aust Crit Care* 2000; 13:10-13 (evidence level: B)

References – Management of Tunneled Catheter Infection

1. Passerini L, Lam K, Costerton JW, King EG. Biofilms on indwelling vascular catheters. *Crit Care Med* 1992; 20:665-673 (evidence level: B)
2. Marr KA, Sexton DJ, Conlon PJ, Corey GR, Schwab SJ, Kirkland KB. Catheter-related bacteremia and outcome of attempted catheter salvage in patients undergoing hemodialysis. *Ann Intern Med* 1997; 127:275-280 (evidence level: B)
3. Capdevila JA, Planes AM, Palomar M, Gasser I, Almirante B, Pahissa A, Crespo E, Martinez-Vazquez JM. Value of differential quantitative blood cultures in the diagnosis of catheter-related sepsis. *Eur J Clin Microbiol Infect Dis* 1992; 11:403-407 (evidence level: B)
4. Nassar GM and Ayus JC. Infectious complications of the hemodialysis access. *Kidney Int* 2001; 60:1-13 (evidence level: C)
5. Schwab SJ and Beathard G. The hemodialysis catheter conundrum: hate living with them, but can't live without them. *Kidney Int* 1999; 56:1-17 (evidence level: C)
6. Kessler M, Canaud B, Pedrini MT, Tattersall JE, ter Wee PM, Vanholder R, Wanner C. European Best Practice Guidelines for Haemodialysis (Part 1) *Nephrol Dial Transplant* 2002; 17 (Suppl. 7)
7. Beathard GA. Management of bacteremia associated with tunneled-cuffed hemodialysis catheters. *J Am Soc Nephrol* 1999; 10:1045-1049 (evidence level: B)
8. Rello J, Gatell JM, Almirall J, Campistol JM, Gonzalez J, Puig de la Bellacasa J. Evaluation of culture techniques for identification of catheter-related infection in hemodialysis patients. *Eur J Clin Microbiol Infect Dis* 1989; 8:620-622 (evidence level: B)
9. Almirall J, Gonzalez J, Rello J, Campistol JM, Montoliu J, Puig de la Bellacasa J, Revert L, Gatell JM. Infection of hemodialysis catheters: incidence and mechanisms. *Am J Nephrol* 1989; 9:454-459 (evidence level: B)
10. Robinson D, Suhocki P, Schwab SJ. Treatment of infected tunneled venous access hemodialysis catheters with guidewire exchange. *Kidney Int* 1998; 53:1792-1794 (evidence level: C)
11. Shaffer D. Catheter-related sepsis complicating long-term, tunneled central venous dialysis catheters: management by guidewire exchange. *Am J Kidney Dis* 1995; 25:593-596 (evidence level: B)
12. Oliver MJ, Callery SM, Thorpe KE, Schwab SJ, Churchill DN. Risk of bacteremia from temporary hemodialysis catheters by site of insertion and duration of use: a prospective study. *Kidney Int* 2000; 58:2543-2555 (evidence level: B)
13. Butterly DW and Schwab SJ. Dialysis access infections. *Curr Opin Nephrol Hypertens* 2000; 9:631-635 (evidence level: C)
14. Tanriover B, Carlton D, Saddekni S, Hamrick K, Oser R, Westfall AO, Allon M. Bacteremia associated with tunneled dialysis catheters: comparison of two treatment strategies. *Kidney Int* 2000; 57:2151-2155 (evidence level: B)
15. Vijayvargiya R and Veis JH. Antibiotic-resistant endocarditis in a hemodialysis patient. *J Am Soc Nephrol* 1996; 7:536-542 (evidence level: B)
16. Kovalik EC, Raymond JR, Albers FJ, Berkoben M, Butterly DW, Montella B, Conlon PJ. A clustering of epidural abscesses in chronic hemodialysis patients: risks of salvaging access catheters in cases of infection. *J Am Soc Nephrol* 1996; 7:2264-2267 (evidence level: B)
17. Kikuchi S, Muro K, Yoh K, Iwabuchi S, Tomida C, Yamaguchi N, Kobayashi M, Nagase S, Aoyagi K, Koyama A. Two cases of psoas abscess with discitis by methi-

cillin-resistant Staphylococcus aureus as a complication of femoral-vein catheterization for haemodialysis. *Nephrol Dial Transplant* 1999; 14:1279-1281 (evidence evel: B)
18. Krishnasami Z, Carlton D, Bimbo L, Taylor ME, Balkovetz DF, Barker J, Allon M. Management of hemodialysis catheter-related bacteremia with an adjunctive antibiotic lock solution. *Kidney Int* 2002; 61:1136-1142 (evidence level: B)
19. Boorgu R, Dubrow AJ, Levin NW, My H, Canaud BJ, Lentino JR, Wentworth DW, Hatch DA, Megerman J, Prosl FR, Gandhi VC, Ing TS. Adjunctive antibiotic/anticoagulant lock therapy in the treatment of bacteremia associated with the use of a subcutaneously implanted hemodialysis access device. *ASAIO J* 2000; 46:767-770 evidence level: B)
20. Nielsen J, Ladefoged SD, Kolmos HJ. Dialysis catheter-related septicaemia - focus on Staphylococcus aureus septicaemia. *Nephrol Dial* Transplant 1998; 13:2847-2852 (evidence level: B)
21. Dobkin JF, Miller MH, Steigbigel NH. Septicemia in patients on chronic hemodialysis. *Ann Intern Med* 1978; 88:28-33 (evidence level: B)
22. Hoen B, Paul-Dauphin A, Hestin D, Kessler M. EPIBACDIAL: a multicenter prospective study of risk factors for bacteremia in chronic hemodialysis patients. *J Am Soc Nephrol* 1998; 9:869-876 (evidence level: B)
23. Kairaitis LK and Gottlieb T. Outcome and complications of temporary haemodialysis catheters. *Nephrol Dial Transplant* 1999; 14:1710-1714 (evidence level: B)
24. Saad TF. Bacteremia associated with tunneled, cuffed hemodialysis catheters. *Am J Kidney Dis* 1999; 34:1114-1124 (evidence level: B)
25. Minga TE, Flanagan KH, Allon M. Clinical consequences of infected arteriovenous grafts in hemodialysis patients. *Am J Kidney Dis* 2001; 38:975-978 (evidence level: B)

References – Appendix

1. Cable DG, Mullany CJ, Schaff HV. The Allen test. *Ann Thorac Surg* 1999; 67:876-877 (evidence level: C)
2. Fronek A and King D. An objective sequential compression test to evaluate the patency of the radial and ulnar arteries. *J Vasc Surg* 1985; 2:450-452 (evidence level : B)
3. Kamienski RW and Barnes RW. Critique of the Allen test for continuity of the palmar arch assessed by doppler ultrasound. *Surg Gynecol Obstet* 1976; 142:861-864 (evidence level: A)
4. Jarvis MA, Jarvis CL, Jones PR, Spyt TJ. Reliability of Allen's test in selection of patients for radial artery harvest. *Ann Thorac Surg* 2000; 70:1362-1365 (evidence level: A)
5. McGregor AD. The Allen test - an investigation of its accuracy by fluorescein angiography. *J Hand Surg [Br]* 1987; 12:82-85 (evidence level: B)
6. Vu-Rose T, Ebramzadeh E, Lane CS, Kuschner SH. The Allen test. A study of interobserver reliability. *Bull Hosp Jt Dis* 1997; 56:99-101
7. Hirai M and Kawai S. False positive and negative results in Allen test. *J Cardiovasc Surg (Torino)* 1980; 21:353-360 (evidence level: B)
8. Ruengsakulrach P, Brooks M, Hare DL, Gordon I, Buxton BF. Preoperative assessment of hand circulation by means of Doppler ultrasonography and the modified Allen test. *J Thorac Cardiovasc Surg* 2001; 121:526-531 (evidence level: B)

9. Levinsohn DG, Gordon L, Sessler DI. The Allen's test: analysis of four methods. *J Hand Surg [Am]* 1991; 16:279-282 (evidence level: C)
10. Fuhrman TM, Reilley TE, Pippin WD. Comparison of digital blood pressure, plethysmography, and the modified Allen's test as means of evaluating the collateral circulation to the hand. *Anaesthesia* 1992; 47:959-961 (evidence level: B)
11. Dousset V, Grenier N, Douws C, Senuita P, Sassouste G, Ada L, Potaux L. Hemodialysis grafts: color Doppler flow imaging correlated with digital subtraction angiography and functional status. *Radiology* 1991; 181:89-94 (evidence level: B)
12. Sapoval MR, Turmel-Rodrigues LA, Raynaud AC, Gaux JC. Upper Limb Venography: Iodine, CO_2. *Dialyse-Journal* 1999; 66:209-210 (evidence level: C)
13. Rieger J, Sitter T, Toepfer M, Linsenmaier U, Pfeifer KJ, Schiffl H. Gadolinium as an alternative contrast agent for diagnostic and interventional angiographic procedures in patients with impaired renal function. *Nephrol Dial Transplant* 2002; 17:824-828 (evidence level: B)
14. Geoffroy O, Tassart M, Le Blanche AF, Khalil A, Ducdal V, Rossert J, Bigot JM, Boudghene FP. Upper extremity digital subtraction venography with gadoterate meglumine before fistula creation for hemodialysis. *Kidney Int* 2001; 59:1491-1497
15. Nyman U, Elmstahl B, Leander P, Nilsson M, Golman K, Almen T. Are gadolinium-based contrast media really safer than iodinated media for digital subtraction angiography in patients with azotemia? *Radiology* 2002; 223:311-318
16. Menegazzo D, Laissy JP, Durrbach A, Debray MP, Messin B, Delmas V, Mignon F, Schouman-Claeys E. Hemodialysis access fistula creation: preoperative assessment with MR venography and comparison with conventional venography. *Radiology* 1998; 209:723-728 (evidence level: B)
17. Hartnell GG, Hughes LA, Finn JP, Longmaid HE, III. Magnetic resonance angiography of the central chest veins. A new gold standard? *Chest* 1995; 107:1053-1057 (evidence level: B)
18. Sands J. The role of color-flow Doppler ultrasound in the management of hemodialysis accesses. *ASAIO J* 1998; 44:41-43 (evidence level: C)
19. Wittenberg G, Schindler T, Tschammler A, Kenn W, Hahn D. [Value of color-coded duplex ultrasound in evaluating arm blood vessels- -arteries and hemodialysis shunts]. *Ultraschall Med* 1998; 19:22-27
20. Malovrh M. Native arteriovenous fistula: preoperative evaluation. *Am J Kidney Dis* 2002; 39:1218-1225 (evidence level B)
21. Bonucchi D, Cappelli G, Albertazzi A. Which is the preferred vascular access in diabetic patients? A view from Europe. *Nephrol Dial Transplant* 2002; 17:20-22 (evidence level: C)
22. Wedgwood KR, Wiggins PA, Guillou PJ. A prospective study of end-to-side vs. side-to-side arteriovenous fistulas for haemodialysis. *Br J Surg* 1984; 71:640-642 (evidence level: A)
23. Polo J, Lago M, Dall´Aneses C, Sanabia J, Goicoechea M, Serantes A. Fístulas radiocefálicas para diálisis. Análisis de una experiencia de 14 anos. *Nefrologia* 1993; 13:313-319
24. Kinnaert P, Vereerstraeten P, Toussaint C, Van Geertruyden J. Nine years´experience with internal arteriovenous fistulas for haemodialysis: a study of some factors influencing the results. *Br J Surg* 1977; 64:242-246
25. Oliver MJ, McCann RL, Indridason OS, Butterly DW, Schwab SJ. Comparison of

transposed brachiobasilic fistulas to upper arm grafts and brachiocephalic fistulas. *Kidney Int* 2001; 60:1532-1539 (evidence level: B)
26. Nazzal MM, Neglen P, Naseem J, Christenson JT, al Hassan HK. The brachiocephalic fistula: a successful secondary vascular access procedure. *Vasa* 1990; 19:326-329 (evidence level: B)
27. Rubens F and Wellington JL. Brachiocephalic fistula: a useful alternative for vascular access in chronic hemodialysis. *Cardiovasc Surg* 1993; 1:128-130 (evidence level: B)
28. Elfstrom J and Lindell A. Limitations of the use of arteriovenous fistulae in the cubital fossa. *Scand J Urol Nephrol* 1994; 28:123-126
29. Piza-Katzer H, Laszloffy P, Schidrich R. Complications of antecubital arteriovenous fistula. *Vasa* 1994; 23:163-166
30. Gracz KC, Ing TS, Soung LS, Armbruster KF, Seim SK, Merkel FK. Proximal forearm fistula for maintenance hemodialysis. *Kidney Int* 1977; 11:71-75 (evidence level: C)
31. Konner K. Increasing the proportion of diabetics with AV fistulas. *Semin Dial* 2001; 14:1-4 (evidence level: C)
32. Polo JR, Vazquez R, Polo J, Sanabia J, Rueda JA, Lopez-Baena JA. Brachiocephalic jump graft fistula: an alternative for dialysis use of elbow crease veins. *Am J Kidney Dis* 1999; 33:904-909 (evidence level: B)
33. Polo JR, Lago M, Goicoechea M, Dall´Agnese C, Serantes A, Sanabia J, Valentín C. Fístulas arteriovenosas para diálisis en el pliegue del codo. *Nefrología* 1993; 13:60-65 (evidence level: B)
34. Barbosa J and Ferreira MJ. Lower Limb A-V Fistulas. *Blood Purif* 2001; 19:117-118 (evidence level: C)
35. Oliver MJ. Acute dialysis catheters. *Semin Dial* 2001; 14:432-435 (evidence level: C)
36. Depner TA. Catheter performance. *Semin Dial* 2001; 14:425-431 (evidence level: C)
37. Level C, Lasseur C, Chauveau P, Bonarek H, Perrault L, Combe C. Performance of twin central venous catheters: influence of the inversion of inlet and outlet on recirculation. *Blood Purif* 2002; 20:182-188 (evidence level: B)
38. Ash SR. The evolution and function of central venous catheters for dialysis. *Semin Dial* 2001; 14:416-424 (evidence level: C)
39. Schwab SJ and Beathard G. The hemodialysis catheter conundrum: hate living with them, but can't live without them. *Kidney Int* 1999; 56:1-17 (evidence level: C)
40. Canaud B, My H, Morena M, Lamy-Lacavalerie B, Leray-Moragues H, Bosc JY, Flavier JL, Chomel PY, Polaschegg HD, Prosl FR, Megerman J. Dialock: a new vascular access device for extracorporeal renal replacement therapy. Preliminary clinical results. *Nephrol Dial Transplant* 1999; 14:692-698 (evidence level: B)
41. Moran JE. Subcutaneous vascular access devices. *Semin Dial* 2001; 14:452-457 (evidence level: C)
42. Schwab SJ, Raymond JR, Saeed M, Newman GE, Dennis PA, Bollinger RR. Prevention of hemodialysis fistula thrombosis. Early detection of venous stenoses. *Kidney Int* 1989; 36:707-711 (evidence level: B)
43. Beathard GA. Percutaneous transvenous angioplasty in the treatment of vascular access stenosis. *Kidney Int* 1992; 42:1390-1397 (evidence level: B)
44. Smits JH, van der LJ, Hagen EC, Modderkolk-Cammeraat EC, Feith GW, Koomans HA, van den Dorpel MA, Blankestijn PJ. Graft surveillance: venous pressure, access flow, or the combination? *Kidney Int* 2001; 59:1551-1558 (evidence level: A)
45. III. NKF-K/DOQI Clinical Practice Guidelines for Vascular Access: update 2000. *Am J Kidney Dis* 2001; 37 (Suppl. 1) : S137-S181

46. Kleinekofort W, Kraemer M, Rode C, Wizemann V. Extracorporeal pressure monitoring and the detection of vascular access stenosis. *Int J Artif Organs* 2002; 25:45-50 (evidence level: B)
47. Turmel-Rodrigues L, Raynaud A, Bourquelot P. Percutaneous treatment of arteriovenous access dysfunction. in: Hemodialysis Vascular Access: Practice and Problems. Conlon PJ, Schwab SJ, Nicholson ML (eds). Oxford, New York Oxford University Press 2000; 183-202 (evidence level: C)
48. Turmel-Rodrigues L, Pengloan J, Bourquelot P. Interventional radiology in hemodialysis fistulae and grafts: a multidisciplinary approach. *Cardiovasc Intervent Radiol* 2002; 25:3-16
49. Beathard GA. Options for restauration of thrombosed vascular access: thrombolysis. Oxford University Press 2000; 203-226 (evidence level: C)
50. Berman SS and Gentile AT. Impact of secondary procedures in autogenous arteriovenous fistula maturation and maintenance. *J Vasc Surg* 2001; 34:866-871
51. Hingorani A, Ascher E, Kallakurl S, Greenberg S, Khanimov Y. Impact of reintervention for failing upper-extremity arteriovenous autogenous access for hemodialysis. *J Vasc Surg* 2001; 34:1004-1009 (evidence level: B)
52. Mickley V, Storck M, Abendroth D. Reversal of blood flow direction for the salvage of forearm straight and looped ePTFE-shunts. *Vasa* 1996; 25:257-260
53. Nassar GM and Ayus JC. Infectious complications of the hemodialysis access. *Kidney Int* 2001; 60:1-13 (evidence level: C)
54. Sarnak MJ and Jaber BL. Mortality caused by sepsis in patients with end-stage renal disease compared with the general population. *Kidney Int* 2000; 58:1758-1764
55. Dobkin JF, Miller MH, Steigbigel NH. Septicemia in patients on chronic hemodialysis. *Ann Intern Med* 1978; 88:28-33 (evidence level: B)
56. Marr KA, Sexton DJ, Conlon PJ, Corey GR, Schwab SJ, Kirkland KB. Catheter-related bacteremia and outcome of attempted catheter salvage in patients undergoing hemodialysis. *Ann Intern Med* 1997; 127:275-280 (evidence level: B)
57. Hoen B, Paul-Dauphin A, Hestin D, Kessler M. EPIBACDIAL: a multicenter prospective study of risk factors for bacteremia in chronic hemodialysis patients. *J Am Soc Nephrol* 1998; 9:869-876 (evidence level: B)
58. Dhingra RK, Young EW, Hulbert-Shearon TE, Leavey SF, Port FK. Type of vascular access and mortality in U.S. hemodialysis patients. *Kidney Int* 2001; 60:1443-1451 (evidence level: B)
59. Schwab SJ, Buller GL, McCann RL, Bollinger RR, Stickel DL. Prospective evaluation of a Dacron cuffed hemodialysis catheter for prolonged use. *Am J Kidney Dis* 1988; 11:166-169 (evidence level: B)
60. Jean G, Charra B, Chazot C, Vanel T, Terrat JC, Hurot JM. Long-term outcome of permanent hemodialysis catheters: a controlled study. *Blood Purif* 2001; 19:401-407 (evidence level: B)
61. Cooper L. The status of access. Is progress being made toward NKF-K/DOQI goals for dialysis access? *Nephrology News & Issues* 2001; 38-45 (evidence level: C)
62. Beathard GA. Management of bacteremia associated with tunneled-cuffed hemodialysis catheters. *J Am Soc Nephrol* 1999; 10:1045-1049 (evidence level: B)
63. Saad TF. Bacteremia associated with tunneled, cuffed hemodialysis catheters. *Am J Kidney Dis* 1999; 34:1114-1124 (evidence level: B)
64. Zaleski GX, Funaki B, Lorenz JM, Garofalo RS, Moscatel MA, Rosenblum JD, Leef

JA. Experience with tunneled femoral hemodialysis catheters. *Am J Roentgenol* 1999; 172:493-496 (evidence level: B)
65. Kairaitis LK and Gottlieb T. Outcome and complications of temporary haemodialysis catheters. *Nephrol Dial Transplant* 1999; 14:1710-1714 (evidence level: B)
66. Schwab SJ, Quarles LD, Middleton JP, Cohan RH, Saeed M, Dennis VW. Hemodialysis-associated subclavian vein stenosis. *Kidney Int* 1988; 33:1156-1159 (evidence level: B)
67. Kovalik EC, Raymond JR, Albers FJ, Berkoben M, Butterly DW, Montella B, Conlon PJ. A clustering of epidural abscesses in chronic hemodialysis patients: risks of salvaging access catheters in cases of infection. *J Am Soc Nephrol* 1996; 7:2264-2267 (evidence level: B)
68. Passerini L, Lam K, Costerton JW, King EG. Biofilms on indwelling vascular catheters. *Crit Care Med* 1992; 20:665-673 (evidence level: B)
69. Fong IW, Capellan JM, Simbul M, Angel J. Infection of arterio-venous fistulas created for chronic haemodialysis. *Scand J Infect Dis* 1993; 25:215-220 (evidence level: B)
70. Zibari GB, Gadallah MF, Landreneau M, McMillan R, Bridges RM, Costley K, Work J, McDonald JC. Preoperative vancomycin prophylaxis decreases incidence of postoperative hemodialysis vascular access infections. *Am J Kidney Dis* 1997; 30:343-348 (evidence level: A)
71. Peleman R.A., Vogelaers D., Verschraegen G. Changing patterns of antibiotic - update on antibiotic management of the infected vascular access. *Nephrol Dial Transplant* 2000; 15:1281-1284 (evidence level: C)
72. Keane WF, Alexander SR, Bailie GR, Boeschoten E, Gokal R, Golper TA, Holmes CJ, Huang CC, Kawaguchi Y, Piraino B, Riella M, Schaefer F, Vas S. Peritoneal dialysis-related peritonitis treatment recommendations: 1996 update. *Perit Dial Int* 1996; 16:557-573
73. Center for Disease Control and Prevention. Recommendation for the prevention of vancomycin resistance. *MMWR* 1995; 44:1-13
74. Marx MA, Frye RF, Matzke GR, Golper TA. Cefazolin as empiric therapy in hemodialysis-related infections: efficacy and blood concentrations. *Am J Kidney Dis* 1998; 32:410-414 (evidence level: B)
75. Musher DM, Lamm N, Darouiche RO, Young EJ, Hamill RJ, Landon GC. The current spectrum of Staphylococcus aureus infection in a tertiary care hospital. *Medicine (Baltimore)* 1994; 73:186-208 (evidence level: B)